The SH!T

NO ONE TELLS YOU ABOUT

PREGNANCY

A GUIDE TO SURVIVING PREGNANCY, CHILDBIRTH, AND BEYOND

Dawn Dais

SEAL PRESS

Seal Press
Hachette Book Group
1290 Avenue of the Americas, New York, NY 10104
sealpress.com
Printed in the United States of America.

First Edition: November 2017
Published by Seal Press, an imprint of Perseus Books, LLC, a subsidiary of Hachette Book
Group, Inc.
The Hachette Speakers Bureau provides a wide range of authors for speaking events. To find
out more, go to www.hachettespeakersbureau.com or call (866) 376-6591.
The publisher is not responsible for websites (or their content) that are not owned by the
publisher.

Editorial production by Christine Marra, *Marra*thon Production Services,
www.marrathoneditorial.org
Set in 9.5-point Sabon

Library of Congress Cataloging-in-Publication Data has been applied for.
LCCN: 2017953114

ISBN 978-1-58005-633-5 (paperback)
ISBN 978-1-58005-634-2 (ebook)

LSC-C

10 9 8 7 6 5 4 3 2 1

To Vivian and Daniel, for destroying my ab muscles
and doubling the size of my heart

Contents

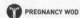
KEY TO EXTRA FEATURES:

 DEAR BEAN LETTER   HOW BIG IS YOUR BABY?   PARTNER CORNER   PREGNANCY WOD

Introduction

W HEN I FIRST found out I was pregnant, I panicked. Mine was about as far as you can get from an unplanned pregnancy (think a romantic encounter with a 65-year-old nurse practitioner wielding a vial of sperm), but I was still scared all the way shitless when faced with the reality of a positive pregnancy test.

As I sat on the floor of my bathroom, surrounded by peed-on pregnancy tests, my body was officially in the process of building another body. When that building was complete, my body was going to expel the new body through the most unfortunately small of exits. Then, after all those Discovery/Sci-Fi Channel shenanigans took place, I was going to be responsible for the well-being of this tiny human I made from scratch.

So I freaked out a little. Because I was officially in over my head.

To calm my panic I immediately bought every book I could find having to do with pregnancy. I piled them on my nightstand, as if being in close proximity to 3,000 pages of gestation facts would somehow make my uterus smarter.

Each night I would pick up one of these pregnancy tomes and begin to flip through it. I had such high hopes of learning all there was to know about my body and the baby it was growing. But I would usually only make it about three pages before falling asleep or swapping the book for a mindless celebrity magazine (sometimes there were pictures of pregnant celebrities in the magazines, so technically I was still doing research).

When I set out to write my own book about pregnancy, I had one clear goal in mind: Do not bore the pregnant women to sleep or to *Us Weekly*. This might seem like an easily attainable goal, but then you might not be taking into consideration exactly how tired pregnant women are or how inviting the pages of *Us Weekly* can be.

I'm not a doctor (as should have been apparent by the word *Sh!t* on the cover of this book). Absolutely nothing I share with you within these pages is in any way based on science or research into science (unless you count hours spent on WebMD as "research into science" [which you should, because I was able to diagnose myself with 35 extremely rare diseases while on there]). But methinks you didn't pick up a book with the word *Sh!t* on the cover in hopes of discovering a detailed look into pregnancy on a molecular level.

What you were most likely hoping to find, and what I have aimed to provide, is an honest look at pregnancy from the point of view of someone who has made her way through two of them. Think of me as your (overly sarcastic) best friend who is not going to let you head into procreation without some advanced warning of what's coming your way.

What do most friends do when you tell them you're pregnant? They usually give you a wholehearted, "Yay!" (or maybe a less-hearted, "Yay?" if they are unclear as to the whether the pregnancy was planned). But I'm aiming to be the friend who immediately sits you down, hands you a pad of paper, and tells you to take some notes, because it's not all going to be gender-reveal parties and funny onesies.

I've also brought along some of my own friends who have their additional notes to share (you might need a bigger pad of paper). I call these friends my "Moms on the Front Lines" (or MOFL) throughout the book. They have been out in the parenting battlefields for years and are reporting back with what they have learned. As you make your way through the various stages of parenthood you will soon realize that mom friends can be just as valuable as doctors (and not only because doctors never offer you wine). Moms are a great resource because they've been there, cleaned that, and are a reassuring reminder that we are all sorta making this up as we go along (with the help of WebMD).

In addition to my MOFL, I've asked some partners (dads and co-moms) to share their point of view. Partners sometimes get lost in the shuffle during pregnancy, but it's a pretty big time in their lives too. So tell yours to grab another pad of paper and pull up a seat.

A big difference between this book and other pregnancy books is that this book not only focuses on your gestation, but also on what is waiting for you on the other side of your delivery, namely that tiny human we spoke of previously. I think pregnancy is a beautiful time in a woman's life (if you don't count all the gross stuff that happens), but more than that I think it is a very important time. Important not only in a "Circle of Life" sort of way, but also in a "Shit Is About to Get Real" sort of way.

As soon as that pregnancy test strikes positive, your count-down clock is started. In a matter of months you will be expected to take a newborn baby into your home and will be left responsi-ble for its survival. I know, that seems more than a little alarming considering the fact that the contents of your fridge are currently 92 percent take-out containers and every plant in your house is 100 percent dead.

For your sake, and mostly the sake of your upcoming child, you need to spend these pregnancy months getting into prime parenting shape. This means less nursery planning, and more building up your tolerance to being in public with poop on your clothes. It's important.

To that end I've littered this book with various ways that you can prepare yourself and your life for Hurricane Baby. There are lists and tips, warnings and advice to help you maximize these precious training months before you are going to need to be ready for action. I've even developed a series of Parenting WOD (Workout of the Day [like CrossFit, but my workouts involve more openly weeping]) to gradually build up your child-rearing reflexes.

Because I like to think of pregnancy as a countdown to par-enthood, I've divided up the chapters of this book into quarters, like a sporting event. A sporting event that involves sprinting through Babies "R" Us, fighting through aches and pains, and catching a number of gifts that are going to be thrown your way by fans. Your team has a lot of work to do before that final buzzer goes off, and it's time to get a game plan in order now.

Whether you are pregnant, thinking about getting pregnant, or weirdly hanging out in the pregnancy aisle of the bookstore, I'm here to make your journey a little more fun and fill it with a lot more truth. I'm going to encourage you through 40 weeks of pregnancy and send you into parenthood armed with every-thing you need to survive (a sense of humor, Post-it notes, and the ability to pick things up with your toes are three of the top necessities).

So many adventures await you on this journey. You'll be horny yet bitchy, tired yet filled with the urge to reorganize every closet in your house, ecstatically happy yet able to uncontrollably sob at the drop of a sappy Internet video. And that's just what an average Saturday night holds in store after that pregnancy stick gives you a thumbs-up.

Let's make a baby!

Moms on the Front Lines

WHEN I FOUND out I was pregnant, I not only ransacked the pregnancy section of the bookstore, I also made efforts to ransack the brains of anyone who had ever grown a baby inside of them. I had questions and the tendency to send an alarming number of those questions via text message at all hours of the day and night.

My friends always answered my texts, no matter the time, and never failed to calm my nerves. They would offer me advice, an ear, and a little perspective. But more than anything they would offer a "You're fine. Everything is going to be fine."

Throughout pregnancy and parenting there is something uniquely comforting about hearing other moms' stories from the front lines and knowing that they survived to tell the tale. Their advice comes from years of trial and (mostly) error, and their calm comes from having already worked their way through the freak-out portion of their parenting program.

I've asked some of my mom friends to join me in this book to offer their advice and their calm. They are my Moms on the Front Lines (or MOFL, as I call them throughout the book) and they've been deeply embedding in the parenting trenches for years. They have over 30 pregnancies to their credit and they are here to share all that they have learned (mostly they've just learned that they should have slept a lot more before having kids).

Pregnancies are like little hormonal, bloated snowflakes— each one different from the other. My MOFL are here to tell you about their unique experiences and hopefully you will be able to connect with bits and pieces of all of them (if nothing else, please connect to the pieces where they recommend you take lots of naps before the baby arrives).

There are a lot of different moms who pop up throughout the book, but these are the names you will see most often. I asked them to introduce themselves and share their favorite and least favorite parts about being pregnant.

ME, DAWN: My partner, Becky, and I have been together about nine years. We have two kids, Vivian, age 6, and Daniel, age 4. My favorite part of being pregnant was feeling their endless kicks. Both of my kids were doing advanced acrobatics in my womb for months leading up to their delivery. It was always a fun reminder that they were in there and this was all really happening. My least favorite part of both pregnancies was the first 20 weeks, when I felt like I was going to vomit 24 hours a day. As far as pregnancy reminders go, I much prefer the kicking over the nausea.

AMY: Married 15 years, we have two girls (8 & 5). I loved the feeling of being pregnant but didn't enjoy it at the time because I kept waiting for the pregnancy to end like so many had previously (Debbie Downer). I also loved that with my first pregnancy I woke up on Mother's Day (six months pregnant) and started leaking milk. The changes in the body are amazing and disgusting all at once! And how can anyone not say that the best part is feeling/seeing that baby move inside you?!

BROOKE: I've been married six years. We have two kids, a 6-year-old girl and a 4-year-old boy. I loved being pregnant both times! Feeling the baby moving/kicking/turning is incredible. My biggest concern was going into labor when my husband was traveling for work and him not making it back in time.

CARRIE: I have been married 10 years and have two boys, 5 and 7 years old. I loved the very different experiences each time I was pregnant. They were complete opposites in the womb and today they still are. Fascinating how their personalities shine right from the start. I loved the day I got to hold them in my arms and finally welcome them to the word. I love being mom to two rowdy boys (most days)!

DANA: I've been married 11 years. We have two kids (girl 6, boy 4). My pregnancies and deliveries were pretty drama free (which is why I'm a little sad we aren't having any more), but the hormone changes are no joke. Especially postpartum . . . you aren't really yourself again until you get to start sleeping consistently (which can vary depending on the child).

KAREN: I am a single mom. My pregnancy was complicated with weekly tests that ended up with me delivering three weeks early and staying in the NICU for two weeks. And my daughter required two blood transfusions. Best pregnancy memory: stretchy pants. Worst memory: knowing my blood was poisoning my daughter in the womb and every week she could get worse. My advice for pregnant women: Take the four weeks off work before the baby is here if you can. It's the last real "me" time you will get for 18 years.

KAYSEE: I have been married 10 years and have three children; one boy and two girls who are now 9, 7, and 4 years old. Each time I am pregnant I love the day you feel the baby kick inside and the day the baby is born and placed in your arms! Being a mother to my three awesome children is the best thing in life!

JEN: I was married six years. My kiddos are now 8 and 6. With both pregnancies I loved the first ultrasound where I actually got to see them. I remember being in tears because it became real. Of course when I could start feeling them, it was the most amazing experience ever! I do have to say nothing beats the first time the doctor put the baby on my chest. Priceless!!!!!! Love my babies . . . they are my reason!!

MELANIE: I've been married 12 years. We have one boy, age 7. My least favorite part of pregnancy were all of the various tests that had results reflecting potential risks/issues. Favorite part was feeling him kick and watching my family react to him kicking, especially my husband and parents.

MICHELLE: I have been married 11 years and have two boys, ages 4 and 6. My favorite part of pregnancy was having a cute round belly. I called it my "belly with a purpose." Only when pregnant is it acceptable to have a ginormous gut! My least favorite part of pregnancy was having gestational diabetes. But I would do it all again if only my husband would agree to a third.

MICHAELA: I've been married 6 years and we have two kids—a boy and girl, 4 and 2 years old, respectively. For sure the moving belly is the best, but I'd add to that announcing each pregnancy to our friends and family (and even my students) was fun. Probably the worst pregnancy memories I have involve going past my due date, gaining a shit-ton of weight, and feeling like there was no end in sight!

SARAH: Married 10 years and we have two boys, 4 and 7. I loved being pregnant. I loved that I was always warm when I was pregnant and I loved feeling them move. My least favorite part was when my water broke because I knew I wasn't ready for them to come out.

STEPHANY: I've been married 11 years and we have one son who just turned 2. My favorite part of being pregnant was feeling Logan moving around so much. He was super active and it was fun to watch my belly bounce around. It also gave me peace of mind. I had a really easy pregnancy (which I feel was well deserved after everything we went through to get him here!), so I didn't really have any least favorite parts. Well, I guess I didn't like my water breaking suddenly because that was so unexpected and it freaked me out. I had been warned in one of my pregnancy classes about a prolapsed cord if your water breaks, and I remembered they told you to lay down if your water broke. So, I was laying on the floor until I realized that I had to get up to go to the hospital.

TARA: I've been married 9 years. We have three kids, a 4-year-old boy and 10-month-old boy/girl twins. My pregnancies were so different, I feel like I have to talk about them separately. The best part of my first pregnancy was feeling the baby move, and how much better ice cream tastes when you're prego. The worst was the constant worry of all that could go wrong. (Maybe that was the special ed teacher in me.) With the twins, the best was seeing them interact with each other during ultrasounds. The worst? Where do I begin? I will have to say it was the last few months in general and being too miserable to enjoy the anticipation of the babies.

The Partners

BABY MAMAS GET a lot of the focus when it comes to pregnancy. Which is fair since, you know, their uteruses are doing a bulk of the heavy lifting (literally). But pregnancy is a very significant time in the life of partners as well. Partners (dads and co-moms) might not be growing the baby on the inside of their body, but once the child pops out, partners are going to be equally responsible for its well-being. Which means this is crunch time for co-parents as well.

I wanted to bring partners into our pregnancy conversation and give them some advice straight from the mouths of others who have survived living with a pregnant woman (this is actually a much more difficult feat than surviving a baby, because pregnant women have much better aim).

I reached out to partners I know, some of them partners of my MOFL and some who I knew would play along with my mildly intrusive questioning. I wasn't sure what to expect because most of the partners I contacted were men. It's tremendously sexist of me that I didn't think men would have much to say on this subject, and I was pleasantly surprised by the heartfelt answers they gave. I initially only asked a few questions, but once I heard what they had to say I asked more, and more.

I think their insight adds a great deal to this book, not only for other partners, but for pregnant moms as well. Sometimes partners feel like their main job is to support their Baby Mama, so they keep their own thoughts, concerns, and stresses to themselves. If you have a partner, the Partner Corners throughout the book could be a good starting point for some really important conversations the two of you should be having along this journey together.

Here is a breakdown of the partners you'll be hearing from. I asked them each to complete the sentence "Pregnancy is . . ." There were mixed results with that exercise.

BECKY: Becky is my partner. We have two kids, ages 6 and 4.

"Pregnancy is the part of a roller-coaster ride where you're ticking up, up, up. Being a parent starts at the top of that ride."

JASON: Jason is divorced from his first Baby Mama and remarried. He has two boys (11 and 13) and a girl (20).

"Pregnancy is exciting, scary, long, short, difficult, and amazing."

JEREMY: Jeremy has been married to my MOFL Michelle for 11 years. They have two boys, ages 4 and 6.

"Pregnancy is the gateway to a life filled with feces, urine, sleepless nights, and lifestyle terrorists." He's kidding. Sort of.

JONATHAN: Jonathan has been married to my MOFL Amy for 15 years. They have two girls, ages 8 and 5.

"Pregnancy is the most exciting/terrifying experience I've ever willfully signed up for."

KEVIN: Kevin has been married for 17 years and has boy/girl twins, age 11.

"Pregnancy is the adventure of a lifetime, every time."

KRISTA: Krista has been married for nine years. She has three sons, ages 6, 20, and 22.

"Pregnancy is an amazing experience. Brewing a human? Miraculous."

MATT: Matt has been married 18 years and has four kids, ages 13, 11, 7.5, and 5. When I asked Matt to complete my "Pregnancy is . . ." sentence he said he was unable to answer, "This is not a good hour. Diarrhea and temper tantrums. Different kids." So, although he didn't answer what pregnancy is, he did a great job describing parenthood.

PETE: Pete is the winner with five kids, including two sets of twins that were born within two years of each other (his kids are ages 16, 16, 14, 14, and 11). He's been married 22 years. I'm assuming he is very tired.

"Pregnancy is a miracle!" When I shared Jeremy's thoughts with Pete he added, "I'm much more of an optimist now that I know we're not having any more!!"

PRE-GAME

1

THE CALM BEFORE THE STORM

50 things you should do before getting pregnant

AVING A BABY is an exciting and wonderful life event. It is also an unprecedented life-changing event. In fact, in the beginning it can feel a lot heavier on change than it does on excitement. This is not to say that change is a bad thing, but having it come on so quickly can be a bit startling.

One day you are free as a (very large, very pregnant) bird, and the next you are functioning on two hours' sleep and responsible for the survival of a tiny human. And I'm not talking about the metaphorical "next day" that people always refer to when describing change that actually takes place over a long period of time. I mean literally you can be napping at 3 in the afternoon one day, having fallen asleep while watching a *Golden Girls* marathon, and *the very next day* you can find yourself holding a newborn baby, everything having gone ass over teakettle.

Again, this isn't a bad thing; the baby is a dream come true! This is a change you (probably) wanted for years, and now it has finally happened! But before it happens I have some things you need to do. Bucket list items, if you will. It's not that you are dying, per se, it's just that your bucket list is soon going to be replaced by a diaper pail. And a lot of your freedoms are indeed passing over to the other side. Or, more accurately, you are passing over to the other side, to the parenthood side of your life. Before you pass, take some time to enjoy the view on this side of things.

Pre-pregnancy you are a lot like the free bird I spoke of earlier. You can fly where you want, when you want. Nothing is holding you back (and the things you think are holding you back are really just figments of your imagination). And then you have a baby, and all of a sudden you are nest-bound for the foreseeable future. It's not that you don't love your baby, or your nest, but you do miss the flying. And you realize that you didn't truly appreciate the flying when it was so readily available to you.

My MOFL (Moms on the Front Lines) are baffled at the amount of free time they wasted before their kids arrived: "I laugh that I used to say I didn't have time for the gym or to take up a hobby or read a book. What was I doing that I thought I was so busy? I had nothing but time!"

Jen recommends appreciating your free time at restaurants: "Eat out at restaurants . . . and linger!"

Ah, to linger.

When I asked my MOFL to pass along their advice to people who have yet to have children, they all collectively screamed "travel!" and "sleep!" at the same time.

"Travel, travel, travel."

"Definitely travel more. Overseas, if you can swing it."

"Travel, even if it is just for the quick weekend trip. And when you do, enjoy only packing a small suitcase."

"S L E E P."

"Go on vacation and sleep."

Might I recommend sleeping through an entire vacation?

Dana, mom of two, wishes she traveled more, but didn't think they had enough money at the time. Amy thought she was broke too, but had no idea how much disposable income she was sitting on, "I thought I didn't have any money to travel, but then we somehow managed to come up with $1,000 a month for daycare?!"

Sarah seconded that motion, "Seriously, Amy!! Think of all the places you could go with the money we spend on daycare, diapers, and food!!!"

My MOFL would like you to know that, pre-children, you are flush with freedom and cash, apparently.

Now, I'm not saying that traveling the world or embarking on the ambitious goal of incorporating siestas into your daily routine pre-kids is going to make your time as a parent a delightful exercise in peace and contentment. In fact, all that bucket-listing might just make you acutely aware of what you are missing once that child puts an end to all things adventure.

For instance, I knew I wanted to have kids in my early thirties. Therefore I made it my mission to have as many exploits as possible before that time. Among other things, I rode my bike across Europe, took an eight-week road trip throughout the United States, drove a car around Cuba with no map (or Spanish), led Habitat for Humanity trips to New Orleans, and jumped off questionable cliffs in Honduras. I saw theater on Broadway, quit a safe job and took a chance on new career, trained for a marathon, and ate the majority of my meals in nice restaurants. Oh, and I slept a hell of a lot too.

Even with those deliberate attempts to fit everything in before having kids, I still regularly feel the tinge of missing all the freedom (and rest) I once had. But I'm so glad I had all those adventures, and I love telling my kids about them, hopefully planting seeds for their own future bucket lists. And as I get older I realize that there are few truer quotes than "Twenty years from now you will be more disappointed by the things that you didn't do than by the ones you did. So throw off the bowlines. Sail away from the safe harbor. Catch the trade winds in your sails. Explore. Dream. Discover." And also, you know, nap.

And so I've created a list of things you should do before you even get pregnant, when you are still in full bird of freedom mode. If you didn't pick up this book until you became a pregnant bird, that's okay; a lot of this stuff can be done with a child in your uterus. I've marked a (p) next to the line items that are probably off-limits once you're with child, but conveniently most of those will come back into play a little while after the kid makes an appearance, so don't get too worked up over them.

I've also allowed space at the bottom of the list for you to fill in a few bucket items of your own. So you can add that thing or place or nap location you've always wanted to try.

Happy flying, little birds!

50 *Things to Do Before Getting Pregnant*

1. Nap at 2 PM on a Sunday
2. Or any day, really
3. Do absolutely nothing when you get home from work. Nothing.
4. Order an appetizer at dinner

5. Travel alone

6. Stay out past midnight drinking (p)

7. Do nothing the next day to recover from your hangover (p)

8. Read a book

9. Eat raw cookie dough (p)

10. Order dessert at dinner

11. Travel someplace that requires getting shots (p)

12. Watch lots of TV shows and movies with cuss words and gratuitous sex/violence

13. Sleep on your stomach (p)

14. DRINK! (p)

15. Tell your waiter there is no rush

16. Read a magazine from cover to cover in one sitting

17. Say yes when someone asks you to go somewhere at the last minute

18. Eat so much sushi (p)

19. Drink so much wine (p)

20. Eat a deli sandwich (p)

21. Drink a gallon of coffee (p)

22. Eat whatever the hell you want because your body isn't responsible for growing/feeding another body (p)

23. Buy a comfortable king-size mattress

24. Read another book

25. Wear the hell out of that fancy party dress (preferably at a party, but even to the grocery store is acceptable)

26. Go someplace that is decidedly not kid-friendly (perhaps somewhere that requires silence from its

patrons, or has sharp objects in plain view, or has anything of value not nailed down)

27. Skydive (or something else that would be phenomenally stupid to do when you have other people counting on your survival) (p)
28. Binge watch an entire TV series on Netflix over the course of a single weekend because you actually have the time to yourself to do such things
29. Go on a road trip and only stop the car when you want to
30. Take a shower alone
31. Take a poop alone
32. Go to Vegas and spend too much money
33. Go to bed at 7 PM because you are tired and in charge of your own sleep habits
34. Eat sweets while standing in the middle of the kitchen where anyone could see you
35. Stay in bed all day if you are sick
36. Date your spouse
37. Watch an entire sports game without interruption
38. Go to the gym
39. Decide to leave the house, then do so 45 seconds later
40. Go to a beach and lie on it doing nothing
41. Sleep in
42. Have sex
43. Whenever you want
44. Wherever you want
45. As loud as you want

46. For as long as you want

47. You know that place you have always wanted to visit? Go there.

48. You know that thing you have always wanted to try? Try it.

49. You know that thing you have always wanted to do? Do it.

50. Sleep. Just. Sleep.

52. _____

53. _____

54. _____

55. _____

2 HOW BABIES ARE MADE
A refresher course

$\mathcal{I}$F YOU PICKED up a pregnancy book, you are probably already pregnant or you thinking about getting pregnant. There are a myriad of ways that this condition can come about. Let's discuss a few now.

THE OOPSIE

The Oopsie Pregnancy falls into the Less Than Planned category of procreation. Oopsie, my partner and I didn't mean to get pregnant at this time. Oopsie, I forgot to use birth control (or forgot that birth control is not always effective). Or Oopsie, this relationship was never supposed to last more than a couple of weeks and now has extended its run for about 18 years. The Oopsie Pregnancy is its own unique undertaking and I've undertaken it in its own special chapter—Chapter 3: "Pregnancy Doesn't Always Have Time to Hear About Your Plans. *How to embrace your Oopsie.*"

THE OLD-FASHIONED WAY
(If they used ovulation predictor kits in the olden days)

Some couples decide they are ready for babies and it's a pretty easy equation. They throw out their birth control pills and condoms and start stockpiling *What to Expect* books and gender-neutral onesies. Bring on the gestation!

They may try the popular "Have a Crazy Amount of Sex" method (men are particularly fond of this method), or they may go the slightly more scientific route of tracking ovulation. Tracking ovulation involves the woman having to pee on her hand quite a bit (while peeing on an ovulation tracking stick a little bit). The couple will start planning their sex life around said ovulation, so that urinating on a hand will become a standard part of foreplay. Which is super sexy.

Men are less fond of this method because all the "making a baby" sex they were promised mostly just consists of their partner running at them with an ovulation stick, demanding use of a penis. It's not quite the lingerie and lustful encounters they had imagined when they signed up for this.

CALLING IN REINFORCEMENTS

For some people it can very quickly begin to feel like their bodies didn't get the memo that egg fertilization is supposed to be simple. In fact, as months and months of unprotected sex produce nothing more than a pile of negative pregnancy tests, couples can develop an increasing desire to smack the hell out of their high school health teacher for making it seem as though pregnancy was something that could accidently happen.

Even sexier than ovulation stick foreplay is what happens if attempts at home fertilization don't work and medical personnel are called in to help. Because nothing says an intimate act of love between two committed partners like jerking off into a cup or getting dye shot up into your ladybits. Isn't nature wonderful?

Once doctors get involved in making a baby the road can get a little more bumpy and a lot more frustrating. Medical intervention can range from simple fertility medication to IUI (injecting sperm into a primed uterus) or IVF (mixing sperm and egg together and injecting a fertilized egg into said uterus). All these options turn what is supposed to be a natural act into a big orchestrated science experiment. And it turns out science experiments are a lot more expensive and cause a lot more alarming hormone levels than natural acts.

But the good news is, I'm not sure there is a better precursor to the realities of parenthood than spending a boatload of money while battling mood swings and overwhelming feelings of incompetence. So those on the infertility track are really just getting a jump on things, if you think about it.

PREGNANCY AFTER INFERTILITY

If you successfully get pregnant after infertility or even pregnancy loss (see Chapter 6: "Sometimes It All Goes to Shit. *Surviving a miscarriage*"), you might not have the same level of excitement that other women have throughout their pregnancies. It's not that you aren't happy, it's that your happy is weighed down by a healthy dose of fear. Yes, you finally got pregnant, but there are so many things that could still go wrong. And your struggles this far have conditioned you to expect things to go wrong, because so many already have.

There is nothing I can tell you that will magically lift this fear, and it very well might linger right up until you hold your baby for the first time. But I do encourage you to allow some excitement in as well. Let yourself peruse the baby section of Target. Pick up the tiny newborn outfits and imagine your baby filling them out. As you get into your second and third trimesters, start planning that nursery and let your friends throw you the best baby shower ever. Lean into the joy of these months, even if that joy is always tempered by a little fear.

Also, you may feel guilty if you don't love every second of this pregnancy you worked so hard to create. You may hesitate to bemoan your morning sickness, or swollen ankles, or uncontrollable passing of gas. All of these side effects are part of something you not only signed up for, but spent quite a bit of time (and maybe money) trying to make happen.

But I say, lean into the bitching as well. You've worked hard to get here, you've more than earned your right to complain. If you are having trouble in this particular area, you've definitely come to the right book—you will find plenty of lessons in bitching throughout the following pages. Let me guide you the way.

HOW TO BE A GOOD OLD-FASHIONED PREGNANT PERSON

If you are lucky enough to get pregnant the Old-Fashioned Way, odds are you know at least one person who isn't having such an easy time getting her uterus on board with her procreation plans.

You may feel awkward around this person because you know your pregnancy might be a bit of a slap in the face to someone who is struggling with fertility.

I asked one of my MOFL, Stephany, who had fertility issues for over seven years, if there was anything she would have liked her pregnant friends to know during that time, "I was always grateful when people texted or emailed to let me know they were pregnant. It was easier to absorb it that way rather than being completely taken off guard by a phone call or in-person conversation. That way when I talked to them in person, they were only seeing me being happy for them and not the sadness I felt for myself."

Stephany also had thoughts on whether she liked being included on the invite list for baby/kid events during those tough years, "I think people should keep their childless friends in the loop. Still invite them to baby showers, kids' birthdays, etc. Let them decide if they feel like going, but leaving them out just increases the feeling that something is wrong with them and everyone is leaving them behind. Infertility is already a very lonely process for a couple, so they don't need more isolation."

IF YOU AREN'T ALREADY PREGNANT

First of all, if you aren't already pregnant and you are reading a pregnancy book, there is a very good chance you are a planner. I enjoy a planner. I can't wait for all the highlighting that you are going to do to the pages of this book.

Second of all, in the spirit of planning I have some advice. Doctors will tell you to give the Old-Fashioned Way a solid

12-month effort before seeking out medical help on your pregnancy journey. But I think that is rubbish. That would be like waiting 12 months to go get a broken leg checked out, because you never know if maybe it'll just fix itself.

If you are planning on getting pregnant, you are planning on having your body make another body. I say it might be a solid idea to get your body checked out before taking on that particular task. So, as soon as you start thinking you might want to start thinking about procreating, pay a visit to your general practitioner. Then start tracking your ovulation using either ovulation sticks or, better yet, a fertility monitor. A monitor is more expensive, but it gets to know your cycle and can be very accurate in telling you exactly when you are fertile. You'll need to track your cycle for a couple of months so that you can get a clear idea how your body operates.

Then you need to make an appointment with a fertility doctor. Tell them you are a lesbian or single if you have to, so they will see you before the standard 12 months of infertility. Best-case scenario, they send you off with a clean bill of health and an assurance that your uterus is in prime baby-making shape. And worst-case scenario, they find something that could impede said baby-making. But wouldn't it be great to have that info before you waste 12 months peeing on ovulation sticks?

No matter how your particular pregnancy came/comes to be, I'm so glad this book gets to be part of your exciting ride ahead. This ride has ups (first ultrasound!) and downs (first time puking in a public toilet!), twists (gender reveal!) and turns (so many hormones!). And at the end you will be handed a tiny person who you must raise to be a contributing member of society. Sure, this all may sound a little more like Tower of Terror than It's a Small World, but that doesn't mean we can't have a little fun along the way. So buckle up, hold on, and get ready for the ride of your life.

Dear Bean Letters
Week 5, The Beginning

I've scattered letters throughout this book that I wrote to my first baby, Vivian, while I was pregnant with her. We gave her the nickname "Bean" early on in my pregnancy, because that was how big she was according to my pregnancy tracker at the time. These "Dear Bean" letters will give you a little insight into my first pregnancy and will also someday serve as a reminder to my daughter about exactly how much I went through to bring her into this world. I'm only including letters that I wrote during my first pregnancy because (1) I'm assuming most of my readers are first timers as well, (2) no one has the energy to write introspective letters during their second pregnancy, and (3) if they did, the letters would go something like this: "Week 12—Growing a placenta is still really hard. Why won't this other child let me nap?"

Dear Bean,

I've decided to start keeping a little journal throughout your pregnancy. To write you letters to keep you apprised on how things are going on this side of my belly. We don't know yet if you are a boy or a girl, so I'll just address the letters to Bean, because that is what we have started calling you. My pregnancy tracker says that's how big you are. I'm not sure if we will eventually call you watermelon, but I'm not ready to think about that visual just yet.

Oh, where to start? I would say that we should start at the beginning, but where is your beginning, exactly? Most might assume that your story began the day you were made, when sperm met egg. But I think we have to go back further than that. Because the day you were made was just one more day along your windy road to being.

If I had to pick a beginning of your story, it would probably be way back before pregnancy was even considered. When Mama and I started talking about having a kid, the conversation centered on adoption. We met with the lawyer, took the required classes, passed the home visit, and printed up quite a few of our Dear Birthmother letters.

The letter itself was actually a large pamphlet containing pictures and information about Mama and me. We described our home, our hobbies, our pets, our family and friends. We took lovely photos and I used my graphic design skills to make the pamphlet pop with color and the warmth of visual hierarchy. I was hoping that this extra attention to design would help make up for the fact that we were two women and most birth moms were probably looking for the perfect husband and wife to raise their unborn child.

Apparently my design didn't dazzle because we never got picked. This broke our hearts. The waiting around for someone else to deem us acceptable to parent was frustrating and more than a little humbling. I grew impatient and sad. I impulsively brought home three foster kittens from a pet store one day, because I so needed a baby something to shower attention upon. I randomly decided I was going to make a movie, because I wanted to take on a project that I had some control over. I spent hours online reading other couples' Dear Birthmother letters and convinced myself that each and every one of those couples had more to offer a child than us.

It wasn't the best of times.

For some reason I'd always imagined adoption as the way I would become a mother. I'm not sure why, exactly. I'd like to say the reason was a selfless one, that there are babies who need love and I have love to give, so it seemed like a perfect fit. But although that was definitely a perk of my plan, I'm guessing that my fear of childbirth is what influenced most of my inclination toward adoption. I was all for someone else doing the gnarly pregnancy and birthing part of the baby-making, while I took the hand-off after the snap and ran the child the rest of the way.

When months and months passed without any offers to hand us off a baby, we began discussing the fact that we actually had not one, but two, functional uteruses at our disposal. Perhaps it was time to take one of them for a spin.

In particular, mine was deemed the best one for the job. See, Mama has diabetes and there is a movie called Steel Magnolias that, among other much more uplifting plot points, includes the story of a diabetic woman who dies because of the ill effects of pregnancy on her body. This movie came out when I was 11 years old and stayed with me for decades to come. Although I was terrified of growing and birthing a baby, I knew that it would be more than a teeny bit selfish to ask Mama to compromise her health because I didn't like the idea of pushing a watermelon out of my whooha.

In essence you can thank Julia Roberts for the fact that you ended up with my DNA.

Since we were heavy on uteruses and light on sperm, we had to figure out how to best go about acquiring that important part of the equation. Off to the sperm bank we went.

Unfortunately, a sperm bank is not like a money bank in that it's not possible to just stop by and pick up a withdrawal at the ATM. I know, I was disappointed too.

To pick up our withdrawal, we first had to make our most important decision to date: selecting what sperm to use. Each man who donates to the bank (also not via ATM, thank goodness) completes a questionnaire and an in-person interview. We were able to scan through hundreds and hundreds of questionnaires, looking for one that magically encompassed everything we were looking for in half of our child's DNA. No pressure.

We initially narrowed the choices down to white men, because Mama is white. And we wanted someone over 6 feet tall, because Mommy is short. Beyond that Mama was looking for education and I was looking for a man who could fill out a questionnaire in a coherent manner. I was also looking for a man who didn't believe that "I play Frisbee golf" was an acceptable answer to a question about athleticism.

As you may or may not have guessed, we were able to weed out a lot of men right off the bat.

Many of the candidates were young. They were "donating" because it was a very easy gig and they could make some extra cash while going to college (or between rounds of Frisbee golf). In reading their profiles I came to realize that young men may produce great sperm, but they don't always have the ability to string thoughtful sentences together at ease.

Mama and I read and read and read. We each saved profiles that we liked, out of the hundreds available to us. It seems like it would be nearly impossible to do, but as we both narrowed down the possibilities, one profile stood out to both of us. Out of all those profiles we each gravitated toward one in particular.

What was so special about this guy? It's hard to say. He just felt different. He was older, first of all, in his late 30s when he donated. And you could hear his maturity in his answers. He was married, and he and his wife were struggling with infertility themselves. You could hear that too. He understood where the people reading his questionnaire were coming from. He appreciated what he was giving to them, and he seemed honored to help.

He was smart—I could tell by his writing. He was thoughtful and had much more thorough answers than other donors. He had been raised Mormon, just like Mama. And he had left the church at a young age, when its values didn't line up with his own, just like Mama.

More than anything he sounded like a man in his responses, whereas most of the other donors sounded like boys. Because most of them were.

He was white, tall, smart, and could string a sentence together! He was our guy!

Once we picked our donor, we then had to decide how to best get him involved in the plan we had for my uterus. The most logical option would be to do an IUI in a doctor's office. But Mama wanted to try the time-honored Turkey Baster Method at least one time at home. Since the sperm bank is about an hour away, this method involved a few moving pieces. I had to track my ovulation, and as soon as my fertility monitor gave me a happy face (a fertile face, maybe?), I had to call the sperm bank and tell them I was fertilely heading their way. They prepped Baby Daddy in a nice nitrogen tank for safe transport. Baby Daddy came in a vial that was about an inch and a half tall and a quarter of an inch in diameter; the nitrogen tank he sat in was about two feet tall and eight inches in diameter. It felt a bit excessive. And yet, after I picked up the tank, I put him in the front passenger's seat and strapped a seatbelt around him to keep him safe on the drive home. I may or may not have even talked to him a little.

Thank goodness, I wasn't pulled over; I can only imagine the holding cell I would probably still be sitting in for being in possession of questionable materials.

Unfortunately, despite my safe (and talkative) transportation of our nitrogen sperm, the Turkey Baster Method did not prove successful. So we officially removed any semblance of normal baby-making and headed to the doctor's office for insemination.

Some people get pregnant after a few glasses of wine and some sexy lingerie. We got pregnant in a room with fluorescent lighting by a kind gray-haired woman with the last name that was strikingly similar to the word "crotch." I found this more than a little entertaining as I lay with my legs up in the air for several minutes after Crotch was done with my crotch.

We figured it would take a few rounds of IUI to get pregnant, because nothing on this journey had been quick. So when I appeared to start my period a couple of weeks after visiting Crotch, we were disappointed but not surprised. But then I realized that the period didn't seem normal, and I Googled "spotting" and "pregnancy" and saw that the two can come together. I didn't tell Mama, but I did take a pregnancy test. Or four.

And what do you know? Each test gave me a big ol' PLUS sign. I immediately ran out of the bathroom and shoved my urine-soaked sticks in Mama's face. She screamed, I screamed. We were so excited.

And so here we are. And there you are. A teeny-tiny little bean in my belly. Your journey is just beginning, and yet I feel like you've already been on such a trek to get here.

At the end of the sperm donor questionnaire, the men are asked if they have any message for the people using their sperm. Our guy said, "Hold 'em and love 'em forever, no matter what." It made me cry when I read it. It still makes me cry when I think about it.

We've waited so long to hold you, but I feel like we've already loved you forever. I can't believe we'll finally get to meet you in a matter of months.

Let's not discuss your method of arrival yet, okay? I'm going to bask in this happy for a while before falling into my month-long panic attack about your delivery.

Yay, baby!

1ST QUARTER
(1–10 weeks)

Your Pregnancy Week by Week

Pregnancy books and apps like to help you visualize the size of the person growing inside you by comparing your baby to an everyday object, like a lovely piece of fruit, such as a pineapple. Everyone knows how big a pineapple is, and this is thought to be helpful and exciting. But it can also be slightly disconcerting.

As a woman inches toward the end of pregnancy, these apps take no mercy on her fragile psyche. A pineapple? Really? How is that spiky visual helping anyone? When I first saw the picture of a pineapple in my pregnancy app, I threw my phone across the room and huddled in bed, trying to get the image of birthing that prickly baby out of my head. I still shudder at the thought.

These fruit and vegetable metaphors can also be confusing. If you are anything like me, they will leave you having to exit the app and Google, "How big is a kumquat?" I mean, I know pregnant women are supposed make a lot of sacrifices for their baby, but adding Swiss chard to my vocabulary is where I drew the line.

I understand the struggle of those of you who frequent a fast-food drive-thru a little more often than a farmers' market. That is why I have come up with a more relatable way to understand the size of your growing rutabaga. Throughout this book I will keep you updated on the size of your fetus by providing you with visuals that are much more relatable than Swiss chard and friendlier than a pineapple.

My pregnancy app once told me that my child was the length of a stalk of rhubarb. I had no idea what rhubarb is, except that it was somehow connected to pie. Now, that's a food I can relate to. In fact, if you were to tell me my baby was as big as a pie, not only would I have an instant understanding of size, but I'd also be happy. Because who doesn't like visualizing dessert?

So that's what we are going to try to do. Give you visuals that make you smile, not ones that send you either looking for a dictionary or a safe place to hide your poor, unsuspecting vagina. We are really doing the Lord's work here, I know.

 Your Pregnancy Week by Week

HOW BIG IS YOUR BABY?

WEEKS 1–4

You don't even know you are pregnant yet, so I'm not going to bother telling your how big your baby is. Suffice to say, it's teeny, teeny tiny (yes, that's a scientific term). In the meantime, why don't you go back to visualizing pie. To help with the visualization, maybe find one to eat.

Partner Corner
WE'RE PREGNANT!

MATT: "I think my wife left a pregnancy test out for me to find. I might've tasted my lunch twice that day. I do remember thinking this is the greatest and most terrifying thing to ever happen to me."

BECKY: "I was so excited. Having a baby completed all of my dreams for the life that I had wished for since I was a kid."

JEREMY: "I remember it like it was yesterday (cue: cheesy sitcom flashback):

"I walked in the door, I noticed the kitchen smelled strongly of pee (which I later reasoned was due to the fact that she had danced around the house with a 'pee wand' in celebration for a long while). It didn't take long before Michelle thrust the stereo-typical little white stick in front of me with a definitive blue line. There wasn't one emotion, but a flood of many that all at once struck me dumb. Anxiety, excitement, worry, fear, happiness, and even a little resentment flooded in. The resentment was a pretty natural response now that I think about it, but a feeling no one talks about. I enjoyed the life we had. The fun, the travel, the two of us. I'd worked hard for almost 30 years to get to this point and now it was going to change. 'Is it gonna change for the bet-ter?' 'I don't like change, change is hard.'

"The anxiety/fear/worry was of course for the unknown. Thoughts like: 'Oh, fuck, this is really gonna happen?' 'What if the baby isn't normal?' 'What if it dies?' 'Fuck! We don't have enough money! (Pro tip: You never have enough money.)'

"I felt excitement and happiness too, of course, because this is what we wanted and what we were trying for. I remember thinking: 'Hell, I didn't know it actually worked! (I always kinda wondered.)'"

KEVIN: "I was ecstatic and scared to death at the same time, because of how hard it was for her to get pregnant. I'm generally a very positive person, but because her pregnancy was difficult from the beginning, it was hard to ignore the possibility that something could go wrong at any time. Finding out we were expecting twins made me more excited and more anxious at the same time."

3

PREGNANCY DOESN'T ALWAYS HAVE TIME TO HEAR ABOUT YOUR PLANS

How to embrace your Oopsie

CHAPTER 2 *How Babies Are Made* touched on how hard it can be for some people to get pregnant. Attempts at impregnation can fail for years and years, despite countless fertility tips and tricks, doctors, and turkey basters.

As if repeated failure isn't frustrating enough, people will constantly (like, *constantly*) hear stories of others who "accidentally" got pregnant. Stories of women who "just walk past their husband and get knocked up." Or "We only had sex one time and I ended up pregnant!" People who are struggling with fertility just love hearing all these stories of accidental impregnation (just *love*).

But for every "Shit, the pregnancy test is negative!" there are just as many "Shiiiiiiiit, all those pregnancy tests are positive!" Because pregnancy tests tend to bring on a lot of strong emotions, one way or another.

An Oopsie pregnancy can be a lot of things. Maybe you got knocked up while in a relationship that was never meant to be long term, maybe you got knocked up when you were younger than you would have liked, maybe you decided to have one last romp with your ex (seriously, don't do this; I can't tell you how many pregnancy stories start this way), maybe you were married, but kids (or more kids) weren't part of the plan right now, maybe you should have paid more attention in those sex ed classes.

However you happened upon your Oopsie, here you are. Surrounded by a pile of positive pregnancy tests. And the inability to drink copious amounts of alcohol to cope. Oh, shit.

First, you need to breathe. Lots of breathing. Sit down on the floor for a minute (or a couple of hours) to make the breathing easier. Probably throw in some crying and a creative assortment of cuss words. Maybe take a few more pregnancy tests, juuuuust to be sure.

Repeat this freak-out for approximately a week. Then get your shit together and get going on a game plan.

One of the biggest things you'll learn throughout parenting is that you are at the absolute mercy of these tiny people you have brought into the world. All attempts by you to control the situation will be met with maniacal baby laughter and perhaps some spit-up, to really bring home the point. Most parents aren't faced with this new reality of total-lack-of-control until their baby arrives. But you, owner of an Oopsie pregnancy, are made aware right out of the gate. Look at you, ahead of the game!

When we were trying to get pregnant the first time via IUI, I didn't think we'd be successful as soon as we were. Also, I wasn't so good at counting. So we ended up having our first child on March 16. My partner is a CPA, and March 16 is pretty much the busiest time of year for her. It was just a splendid time to bring home a newborn baby. Just splendid.

I know that a scheduling conflict is nothing compared to a genuine sit-on-the-floor-of-the-bathroom-in-a-ball Oopsie. But my point is that even when a child is as planned as a lesbian pregnancy has to be planned, there is still room for some "Oh, shit"s. And even when a pregnancy is right on schedule, exactly according to plan, parents still freak out about a myriad of different things. Their freak-outs tend to kick in after the initial excitement, around the time an Oopsie mom is settling into the idea of her pregnancy.

I reached out to a few of my MOFL who have had Oopsies of their own. And they are some of the better Oopsie stories I've heard.

EMILY: "My boyfriend and I had broken up, but we 'hung out' one more time on his birthday. And I ended up getting pregnant. My initial reaction was 'Oh, shit.' I was shocked, scared, worried, and afraid. All those emotions just festered until it really sank in.

"I talked to my boyfriend and he was like, 'It's no problem. We can do this.' It calmed me down a little but I knew it wasn't that easy. I was afraid to tell my parents. Surprisingly they were thrilled and supportive. But they didn't want me to get married just because I was pregnant. That was a hard decision to swallow. I felt like people always looked at my belly and then my ring-less finger.

"My boyfriend and I decided to keep the baby and figured out a way to move forward for her. We didn't end up staying together, but after a lot of bumps and hurdles we now get along really well, for our daughter's sake.

"A baby can change a person's life. It changed mine. It made me a more positive and selfless person. I love being a mom."

KAREN: "I'd just foreclosed on my house and lost my dream job because of the market crash. I found out my boyfriend of over a year was married with an eight-months-pregnant wife. That night I took a pregnancy test and it came up positive. It wasn't a great weekend.

"I sat on my bathroom floor sobbing all night long. I met with the 'boyfriend' the next day and he offered to 'pay to take care of the problem.' I said thank you, but no thank you, and walked away from him. I didn't see him in person for another six years.

"I was in shock and in an 'Oh, shit, what is happening' stupor for a few weeks. Then I decided I could either feel sorry for myself or embrace this new chapter and turn lemons into lemonade.

"My daughter is the best thing that ever happened to me. Every day is difficult and exhausting. People who don't have 100 percent custody of their kids can't understand, and I don't expect them to. I can't imagine my life without my little girl, and after seven years, I wouldn't ever want to go back. She just recently went on a trip out of state with my parents and I couldn't go. Before the trip I was so excited to be unencumbered for five days. I was wrong. I was a basket case and wandered around the house wondering what to do with myself. The day she returned was like the sun shining in my house again!"

SARAH: "We had three kids and we were done. My husband had a vasectomy on Monday, I found out I was pregnant the following Saturday. Honestly, I was pretty sad and angry my entire pregnancy. We'd given away most of our baby stuff. We had just finished a huge remodel and each child finally had their own room. I felt like our family had finally gotten easier, we were out of the baby phase. When I discovered I was seven weeks pregnant with Louie I was in shock! Then I felt very sad.

"My mind never shook that feeling until Louie was born. Then I felt constantly guilty that I hadn't wanted him. He was a beautiful baby! He gave me one last opportunity to have a childbirth the way I wanted (naturally) and I did it!

"Everyone promised me the fourth kid would be a breeze. That proved to be the FURTHEST thing from the truth. Louie was a terrible nurser and we had three months of me nursing 8 to 12 times a day and then pumping 8 to 12 times a day. In addition to all that he had colic until he was four months old. He started crying around 2:30 PM every day (lovely timing, right before the older kids came home from school) and continued to cry until 2 AM every. single. day. for FOUR months. He was such a tough baby!

"But, after the breastfeeding corrected and the colic abruptly stopped, he was AWESOME! I love him so much he makes my heart hurt.

"I'm regularly grateful that God knew our family wasn't done. Louie adds something to our family I can't articulate. He reminds me daily to trust God's plan and not my own. God's plan may not always be the easiest or most logical plan to follow but there is such joy to be found following His path. Louie has been a gift to my family and my faith."

WHETHER OR NOT you believe your Oopsie is God's plan or maybe just a gigantic revision of your well-thought-out life plan,

I hope that my MOFL have helped ease your mind a bit. Emily ended up finding her happily ever after with a single dad and has a great relationship with her daughter's father, Karen's career took off when she accepted a job that was the best fit for single motherhood, and Sarah now has a car that fits six people. Life doesn't always take you exactly where you want it to, but most of the time you'll find that it takes you exactly where you are supposed to go.

Your Pregnancy Week by Week
HOW BIG IS YOUR BABY?

WEEK 5–A SPRINKLE ON YOUR DOUGHNUT
Your baby is the size of just a sprinkle on your doughnut, or one of the handful of sprinkles you ate as a late-morning snack today.

WEEK 6–A BIRTH CONTROL PILL
Your baby is about ¼ inch long, a little bit bigger than the birth control pill you forgot to take last month.

WEEK 7–M&M
At ½ inch, your baby is about the size of an M&M. But decidedly less colorful. You should probably eat a bag of M&M's this week, purely for scientific purposes, of course.

Pregnancy WOD
LIKE CROSSFIT, BUT WITH LESS BATHING

In my 50 Things to Do Before Getting Pregnant list at the beginning of this book (page 3), I mention a lot of things that you should do before the arrival of your child. Most of those things involve napping, relaxing, or generally taking advantage of the fact that you are still the one in charge of your time and sleeping patterns.

And while I do think it's very important to maximize all the wonder of your child-free existence, it is also time to acknowledge that you have a lot of changes coming your way in a matter of months. Not only should you acknowledge these changes, but you are going to need to start preparing for them. On an emotional and physical level.

One of the most difficult aspects of new parenthood is the *new* part. The fact that everything changes overnight and you are left scrambling to figure out how to navigate this new life, which now includes a very needy new person. The scramble is only intensified by your severe sleep deprivation and whack-a-doodle hormones. It's a lot to take on all at once.

But what if you had a handle on parenthood before the baby arrived? What if you not only knew what to expect, but had already built up a skill set to tackle every obstacle? What if you were totally prepared for anything and everything that new little person might throw your way?

Honestly, that's not going to happen. But! That doesn't mean we can't give it a try!

I've designed a nine-month training program to help you ready yourself for the fun that is coming around the bend (and out of your uterus). Inspired by those people who religiously tweet/brag about going to CrossFit, I've developed a series of Pregnancy WODs (Workout of the Day) to get you in prime parenting shape by the time your baby arrives. And the good news is that being in "parenting" shape is about as far as you can get from being in "CrossFit" shape, so I know you are up for the challenge.

CrossFit WODs include exercises like climbing ropes, lifting weights, and running for miles at a time. My Pregnancy WODs (patent pending) focus on much more difficult activities, like decreasing bathing frequency, disrupted sleep, and building up a tolerance for Chuck E. Cheese.

You can take my Pregnancy WOD and do them as many days as you need to feel comfortable with the workout. We will start small and build up to advanced-level parenting by the end of your nine months.

Don't push yourself too hard and by all means don't let your WOD interfere with your very rigorous napping and eating-out-at-restaurants schedule you have going. I mean, let's not get crazy. No matter where you are in your pregnancy, never forget this important mantra: But first, we nap!

Pregnancy WOD
MONTH 1

We are going to start out slow; we don't need you pulling any muscles or having any panic attacks this early in the game. Do the following exercises throughout your first month of pregnancy to loosen up your parenting muscles.

1. Pee while holding a bag of flour.

Back in the day, kids were made to carry around a bag of flour to simulate what it would be like if they had unprotected sex and became teen parents. I'm not quite sure how a bag of flour would disrupt a teen's life in any way that resembles the havoc brought on by a child (besides the fact that both flour and babies tend to leak without warning), but as far as general size and weight goes, flour makes a decent stand-in for a baby. So keep a couple of bags on hand for your WOD each month.

This first exercise is meant to ease you into a small, but significant change in your life post-baby. Once you become a parent, you will all of a sudden have an audience for activities that previously fell into the "private" category. In fact, it's a good possibility that you will give birth with a room full of people staring at your whooha, which is actually a very fitting way to usher in your post-privacy era.

The loss of privacy is not nearly as alarming as you might imagine (the birthing amid a crowd builds up your tolerance pretty quickly), but it can make some of your once solo activities a little difficult from a logistical standpoint. You'll have to use the bathroom, but you are also holding a sleeping/nursing/

>

THE SH!T NO ONE TELLS YOU

needs-to-be-held baby. This will happen regularly, and you will regularly find yourself holding said baby while using said bathroom.

Not only will this strike you as tremendously unsanitary, but it will also be rather difficult to perform the maneuvers required to pull your pants down, sit on the toilet, do your business, get that toilet paper off the damn roll (without unrolling the entire thing), wipe, and pull your pants back up—with just one hand.

Practice this exercise early and often. Once you master using only your right hand, switch and use only your left hand. Repeat. And flush.

2. Have someone tie you to a chair while you hold your bag of flour. Open the bag of flour. Then have the same someone put your cell phone juuuust out of reach on the ground in front of you or on a table beside you. Devise a way to get the phone without spilling the bag of flour.

Yes, there are a lot of challenges that come with parenting a newborn. But none is as great as the challenge you will face when you are holding a sleeping baby and your cell phone is just beyond your reach. MacGyver has nothing on the ingenuity and flexibility of a mom who is on a mission to be reunited with her one source of outside contact. You might as well start stretching those muscles now, so you are ready when it's go time.

Reach your leg out farther than you ever thought you could extend a limb. Devise an elaborate grabbing device, using a remote control, two bibs, a magazine, and your breast pump. Get creative. All this practice will serve you well when this situation inevitably presents itself post-baby.

YOUR BODY IS BASICALLY A SCI-FI MOVIE

4

Special effects include cankles, discharge, bloody gums, peeing all over the place, and unfortunate hair growth

THIS CHAPTER IS about all the wonderful side effects that can come along with growing a human in your uterus.

When I first started gathering a list of all the possible pregnancy side effects, I realized that I'd been told about most of them ad nauseam over the years (especially the one about nausea). And I have no doubt that everyone has already told you about most of the possible pregnancy side effects, too. Or that you've already barreled through every website featuring the topic. So I'm not going to go into great detail about all the different ways pregnancy might accost your body and mind.

The following is a list of some common pregnancy side effects. This is not a complete list, because there are roughly 45,285 ways that pregnancy can wreak havoc on your body.

PREGNANCY SIDE EFFECTS
(from head to (swollen) toe)

Insomnia

Increased hair growth *(not always on the top of your head)*

Vision/hearing changes

Acne

Stuffed-up/bloody nose

Increased sense of smell

Bloody gums

Heartburn/reflux

Nausea

Tender boobs

Growing areolas

Sweaty

Clumsy

Frequent peeing

Increased discharge

Yeast infections

Hemorrhoids

Gassy

Hip and back pain

Leg cramps

Varicose veins

Swelling

Overall super sexiness

And now, since this book is called *The Sh!t No One Tells You,* I'll tell you about the body changes you won't always read about on the mommy blogs.

Suffice it to say, you have quite a few new things happening inside your body now that it is acting as an incubator. Your hormones will be running wild, with HCG, progesterone, estrogen, and relaxin contributing to such fun as aches, nausea, weird hair growth, heartburn, and bloody noses. Some women will hit the pregnancy jackpot and get all sorts of side effects, while others get barely any (we hate these women, and don't like to talk to them).

Here are a few side effects that you may not have heard about just yet. Some are annoying and some can be serious, but all can pop up, so they are worth keeping an eye out for.

Itchy Skin

Many women feel itchiness when they are pregnant and it's not a big deal. It is mildly annoying, but can be explained by the stretching of your skin to accommodate your expanding body. My stomach and boobs were always itchy throughout my pregnancies. It got to the point where putting my hand down my shirt to scratch became something I had no problem doing in public.

But itching can be more than just a minor nuisance (or minor embarrassment, in the case of my hands down my shirt). I've known several woman whose itching was the result of cholestasis, which is a very serious condition that requires you to be monitored by your doctor, and most likely will involve early induction.

Itching and rashes can also be caused by pruritic urticarial papules and plaques of pregnancy (PUPPP). PUPPP is not dangerous to you or the baby, unless you count how annoying it is in its extreme discomfort. But there are a few remedies that can ease your pain once it's diagnosed.

Basically, if you have extreme itching, especially if it's on your hands or feet, let your doctor know right away. There may be something that can be done to help, and your body may be telling you it needs help.

Carpal Tunnel Syndrome

I've only recently heard of carpal tunnel syndrome affecting pregnant women. But, why not, really? Just add it to the list. Fluid retention during pregnancy can cause carpal tunnel syndrome and leave some women with numbness and tingling in their hands. It can also cause shooting pains, which sound fun. I'm sure that they are especially fun in the middle of the night, which is when a lot of women complain of their pregnancy carpal tunnel flaring up.

Again, if you have these pains, let your doctor know. An arm brace may help with your nighttime pain, and will also provide a super-sexy accessory to your nightie.

Depression

Depression during pregnancy is something that isn't talked about much. Postpartum depression gets a lot of attention, but it turns out that many women suffer from the blues during pregnancy as well. This can be really hard for pregnant moms to admit, because they may feel as though they have no right to be sad. But let it be known: With the amount of hormones you have swirling around your body, you have the right to be whatever the hell you want.

Like all kinds of depression, pregnancy depression can get worse if it's hidden away. So if you are feeling depressed or a little blue, talk to your doctor, or even just to your partner. Talk to someone and don't be ashamed of it. There are different options available to help you, and being honest about it will be an important step in the right direction.

Constipation

Constipation is actually a pretty well-known pregnancy side effect, but I mention it because it can lead to other, less obvious issues. One late afternoon when I was pregnant, I started having shooting pains in my stomach. They got so bad I could barely walk. I was in a panic and made an appointment to go see my doctor. I considered going to the ER, because I was sure something horrible was happening. It felt like awful cramping; could it be labor pains? It was way too early for labor. I continued to freak out. Then I managed to walk across the room to the bathroom. Where I went poop. And when I stood up, I was cured of all pain.

So . . . it turns out I wasn't in preterm labor, I was actually just backed up and needed to poop (which you'll find out eventually is very similar to how labor feels, coincidently).

I've known other women who have freaked out over the needing-to-poop pain while pregnant, so stop by the bathroom if you are having weird cramping or bloating. And definitely stop there before you head to the ER in a panic.

Extra Saliva

This is about as insignificant as you can get when it comes to pregnancy side effects, but I spent both of my pregnancies spitting with the frequency of a major-league pitcher who has a lump of chewing tobacco in his mouth. Along with my itching of private areas, random farting, and devouring of potato chips, I would have fit in quite well at a frat house.

WHILE PREGNANCY SIDE effects are very common, don't make the mistake of automatically assuming that it's normal for you to feel miserable. Recently a friend told me about her experience during pregnancy, "I had really bad back pain (couldn't walk) and everyone just thought it was part of the process. It's not! My hips had come out of alignment. I ended up going to an osteopath who put them back into alignment, which was surprisingly not as painful as it sounds! I didn't have to be in pain, but I had to be a hardcore advocate for myself, even with my family."

Most side effects won't be treatable or curable, but they are still worth mentioning to your doctor. You never know what tips and tricks they can offer. Or even spend some time in an Internet wormhole, looking for other women who have experienced the same thing. (Obviously, clear all crazy Internet treatments with your doctor before attempting.) If something feels really off, then follow up with your doctor again, and possibly look for a second opinion if you don't feel like you are being heard.

Occasionally a minor pregnancy side effect can actually be the first sign of a bigger problem, so keep track of all your different symptoms and list them off to your doctor, just to play it safe. You'll want to punch them in the face when they calmly nod their head and say, "Yeah, that's all perfectly normal." But at least you can rest a little easier (albeit, still uncomfortably) knowing that your misery is A-OK from a medical standpoint. And if it's not A-OK, you'll be glad you didn't stay quiet.

Moms on the Front Lines

MIRACLES ARE MESSY

I asked my MOFL for their list of pregnancy woes, and it seems as though gestation is just one big science experiment. One of those messy science experiments that explodes everywhere.

AMY: "I had a super-weak gag reflex. A light breeze against my neck would make me gag. It was how I knew I was pregnant again with my youngest—I put on a necklace and just started gagging nonstop."

SARAH: "I caught so many illnesses and colds when I was pregnant both times. It was like the babies sucked my immune system dry and left me with nothing. I think I was sick every month! I was so happy to be able to take NyQuil again!"

MELANIE: "Swelling!!! Oh so much swelling. My feet were huge early in the pregnancy, like at three months."

ERIKA: "I had cholestasis with my second baby, which causes intense itching (I had scratches all over my belly from itching in my sleep) and can be dangerous for baby. This meant that I had to be induced early, and then it took FOUR FREAKING DAYS to get that baby out! I nearly lost my mind."

RACHEL: "I wet my pants while rocking my daughter to sleep. I assumed it was my daughter who had peed until I got to the bathroom and realized I was soaked, not her. I even had my sister smell my pants to see if it smelled like pee or amniotic fluid in case I was leaking fluid. I called the doctor too. I really didn't think I had peed. But I did. That was rad."

THE SH!T NO ONE TELLS YOU

ELISSA: "I got pretty bad pinkeye both pregnancies. The first kiddo, it was actually my first 'sign.' I got pinkeye and started Googling pinkeye. Then on a whim I googled pinkeye and pregnancy. It's a thing! Within a day or two I took a pregnancy test, and sure enough."

TARA: "Oh, where do I begin . . . let's just go for the kickers . . . PUPPP, which is this horrible itchy rash. I was taking four showers a day using pine tar soap because it was the only thing that brought relief. I'd get up in the middle of the night to take a shower. And as a bonus I smelled like a campfire . . . fun times! And then there is the Bell's palsy. I had, and still partially have, paralysis on the right side of my face. At least I can smile now, but my right eye still doesn't blink."

STEPHANY: "The only weird side effect I had was constantly popping ears. They always felt like I was cupping my hands over them. I had to continuously yawn to try to open them up so I could hear."

MICHELLE: "I had swelling with my first. Not just my legs and ankles, but my face as well. My nose looked ridiculous."

Michelle also had another relatively common pregnancy side effect, gestational diabetes. She is super skinny, has no history of diabetes in her family, and ate well throughout her pregnancy. And yet, she still ended up failing the lovely glucose test they give you to test for diabetes.

The test involves fasting, then heading to the lab, where they make you drink a horribly sweet bottle of liquid and sit in the waiting room for an hour. Then they take your blood. If that test shows that your sugars are too high, then you get to go in and do another, longer test. If you fail that longer test, you officially lose out on the best part of pregnancy— eating whatever the hell you want.

Michelle failed all of these tests and had to alter her diet and exercise from then on out.

"I loved being pregnant until around 26 weeks, when I got diagnosed with gestational diabetes. I had to take the gestational diabetes class, where we learned how to test our blood sugar and eat the proper diet. The funny thing about the class was they gave us a book with portions of food that a diabetic person could eat. There were whole sections crossed out that as a gestational diabetic we weren't allowed to eat. Absolutely no rice, cereal, sugar-free anything. It was frustrating to know that a normal diabetic could eat small portions of most foods, but because I was pregnant I wasn't allowed.

"I couldn't have cake at my baby shower. Normally I hate cake and wouldn't have wanted to eat it anyway. But because I wasn't allowed to have it, I wanted it bad! This hormonal pregnant woman did not take it very well.

"But it did make me even more active, which was a good thing. I would always take a two-mile walk after dinner because it would help keep my glucose number within range."

No cake AND a nightly two-mile walk? Michelle is a much stronger woman than I. Which might explain the overall differences in our bodies post-babies as well. Ahem.

Dear Bean Letters
Week 6, The Wand

Dear Bean,

It turns out I am pregnant. This seems very odd to me. A few weeks ago, I had my legs up in a doctor's office after our IUI, and now I am pregnant. As in, now I am growing a person inside of my body. But it's a very tiny person at this point. So tiny that the doctor can't even see you when using the lovely ultrasound wand that I've become way too familiar with throughout this process.

I always thought of ultrasounds in the way they are depicted on TV. Where women get goo squirted on their belly and a nurse runs a friendly ultrasound device gently over the baby bump. It all looks so carefree on the TV.

But when you are going through fertility testing or you are in the early weeks of pregnancy there is a less than friendly wandlike device that is used for ultrasounds. Calling it a wand makes it sound magical, Harry Potter-ish. But imagine if Harry put a condom and lube on his wand and stuck it up your ladybits. At that point you might develop a different connotation for the instrument.

After several encounters with the wand during my fertility testing, I wasn't particularly looking forward to being reacquainted during pregnancy. But I actually found myself demanding it the other day at the doctor's office.

I had felt some cramping and was scared that I had lost you. Not that I needed cramping to be scared. I'm scared all day every day about your well-being. I take at least one pregnancy test a day to check on you. I know this is crazy, but I can't stop doing it.

When I had the cramping, my crazy notched up a few pegs and I immediately went to the doctor's office. The doctors and nurses were very sweet, and entertained my crazy. They had me take another blood test to confirm I was still pregnant and that my numbers were looking good. They tried to assure me that everything seemed fine.

I demanded they use the wand to look for you. They said you were too little to see with the wand. I demanded they try. So they did. But, as they had warned, we couldn't see you just yet. Although this was to be expected, it most definitely did not help with the crazy.

I left the doctor's office and immediately stopped at the drugstore to purchase another 10 pregnancy tests. The ones I've taken so far tell me that you are okay, or at least that I'm still pregnant.

I've been assured that we will be able to see you at our next appointment in a few weeks. Who knew I would be so excited to see that damn wand again? Let's hope it brings some magic this time.

5

IT'S HARD TO SEE YOUR PREGNANCY GLOW WITH YOUR HEAD IN A TOILET MOST OF THE DAY

When morning sickness is too big to be contained to only one time of the day

N O ONE KNOWS why some women spend some or all of their pregnancies fighting nausea and/or vomiting, while other moms-to-be are blessed with nothing but delightful gestation experiences. But it might have something to do with the fact that the world is a cruel, cruel place.

Morning sickness gets its name because a lot of pregnant women feel the most miserable first thing in the morning. I'm not sure what it's called when you slog through the morning and continue to feel awful all damn day, but I think *f'n bullshit* might be the appropriate technical term.

This bullshit will often sneak up on you just as you are celebrating your new pregnancy. It's all so exciting, there's going to be a baby, aren't we lucky?

Then. It hits.

And you immediately stop feeling lucky. Because lucky people rarely spend this much time face-to-face with a toilet bowl.

Battling nausea and vomiting for your first few months (or all your months, if you're *extra* lucky) can make it really hard to get excited about your pregnancy. It takes a lot of joy out of the experience, because it turns the whole thing into something you are just trying to survive.

"Aren't you so happy about the baby?!"

"Well, right now I'm just trying to not puke all over your face. But I'm sure my euphoria will kick in very soon."

I promise that it will eventually get better. Although I will not say *when* it will get better. Because I was told by my doctor and the Internet that most women started feeling better by week 14. And when that week came and went, it filled me with a rage like no other. How dare the Internet lie to me! Also, some women are sick all the way up until their due date because, as I mentioned earlier, the world is a cruel, cruel place. So hang on (to that toilet bowl), and ride this out. I promise, by week 40 you'll be feeling A-OK.

Meanwhile, there are some tried-and-true methods of minimizing the nausea. I never landed on a cure-all for my all-day morning sickness, despite my constant Google-searching for something magical that could stop the madness. But there were a few helpful go-tos that took the edge off. Here are some things you can try if you too are looking for any possible relief.

Eat constantly: During my second pregnancy I was able to fend off a lot of my nausea by constantly snacking on crackers or something equally bland. If my belly got even a little empty, I started to feel sick. With my first pregnancy I felt sick all the time, whether I ate frequently or not. But because I was so uninterested in food, I did eat a lot of teeny little "meals" (a.k.a.: three crackers) throughout the day, so as to keep myself fed and not to overwhelm my angry stomach.

Buy crackers in bulk and keep them with you at all times, and on your nightstand while you sleep. Throw a few in your mouth to start your day, and continue this culinary treat until you are back in bed again.

Ginger or sour suckers or peppermint: A lot of nauseous pregnant women swear by hard candies, be they ginger or sour or peppermint. I popped all of these and found that the ginger helped a little. I think more than anything, it might just be nice to have a pleasant taste in your mouth; maybe it tricks your body into thinking you feel pleasant everywhere else as well.

Acupuncture: I never tried acupuncture because every time I'd think about scheduling an appointment, I would then think about having to get out of bed and drive to the appointment, and that was just too much of a requirement. But I do have friends who found some relief via needles, so maybe if you can get one to come to your house, it might be worth trying.

Acupressure band: I tried this one, and I felt like maybe it helped, but then I also felt like maybe it just had a placebo effect. Either way, it's a band that you wear around your wrist. It has a button on it that pushes on a pressure point on the inside of your wrist. People wear these to help with motion sickness and some have used them to help with morning sickness as well. Again, I'm not sure how effective they are, but trying them can't hurt! If in doubt, order 12, and line your whole arm with them.

Take a nap, or three: Most of the time burying myself in my bed was the only way I could deal with my morning sickness. Or I guess it was my way of acknowledging that I wasn't up for dealing with anything else. Be gentle with yourself and give yourself time to rest when you feel like crap.

Meds: If your condition gets really bad, your doctor may recommend medication to help you. Keep your doctor in the loop about how you are feeling and what you are able to keep down. They will let you know whether medication is an option worth considering.

I WILL SAY that battling nausea for the first five months of pregnancy allowed me to feel a special kind of euphoria once the misery stopped. I had an appetite again! Good smells smelled good! Food was chewed and swallowed with the abandon of someone who had just been fitted with their first set of dentures! Things like standing up or taking a shower didn't automatically send my body into pre-puke mode! It was amazing how wonderful it felt to just feel normal again.

Another excellent result of prolonged nausea? Your doctor will start recommending that you gain some weight. Never have more beautiful words been spoken than the words "eat more" to a pregnant woman who has just regained her appetite. "I'm on it!" I proclaimed. All you can eat AND a baby! What an exciting time!

Moms on the Front Lines
WORKING THROUGH THE PAIN

I work for myself from home. This meant I was able to spend a lot of time curled in a ball during the particularly miserable pregnancy times. Showering was nearly impossible, and I was rarely able to dry all of my hair without giving up or having to sit on the ground for a half-hour with my head on my knees. So I always wondered how in the hell I would have managed to get it together enough to go into a real job every day. And how quickly I would have been fired for coming to work looking like I'd been run over by a garbage truck.

I asked a couple of my MOFL for their experiences navigating the working world while dealing with all-day morning sickness, and it turns out they are much stronger than I am.

CARRIE: "I had a job in a very 'office environment,' which included meeting with clients while pregnant. I was sick (a.k.a.: on the verge of puking) every day, every hour, for five months straight. It sucked. I kept suckers and crackers and ginger tea at my desk, and that helped take the edge off a little."

KAYSEE: "Morning sickness seemed to get worse with each pregnancy! There were times I would be in my office, and someone would come in to find me in a fetal position on my floor waiting for the sickness to pass. I frequently took naps or slept on the floor in my office during pregnancy! Luckily I had some flexibility. I remember saying, 'This is awful, I will never do this again!' And yet I kept having babies. Once the bundle of joy arrived, I forgot how bad morning sickness was!"

Pregnancy WOD
MONTH 2

Okay, now that we've introduced you to some less taxing exercises (and your bag of flour), we can start adding some mental training as well. At this point in your pregnancy you are still skinny, full of life, and excited about the future. Let's take you down a few notches, shall we?

1. Go to Chuck E. Cheese on a Tuesday night and stay for one hour.

This hour is amateur hour. We are starting small to ease you into the general noise that comes with parenting children. No, you won't be going to Chuck E. Cheese right away with your baby (seriously, don't let anyone convince you to go to Chuck E. Cheese with your baby). But you will be surprised how close your one angry little newborn can get to matching the sound of 100 gleeful kids at Chuck E. Cheese.

2. Pee while holding a bag of flour (and leave the door wide open). When you have friends over.

The door to your bathroom will soon become merely ornamental in your home. You might as well get used to that concept now. Children do not understand the reason for the door, nor do they have any time for your use of it. Eventually you will give in/up and find yourself doing your private business without even thinking about closing the door.

Your houseguests may not be big fans of this development, but now is as good a time as any to prepare them for what to expect when they visit your house post-baby.

3. Sleep for two hours in the nursery rocking chair.

Sleep will become more and more uncomfortable as you get more and more pregnant. But even at its most uncomfortable, pregnancy sleep still allows you to be horizontal when undertaking a slumber. Soon after you bring home baby, you will realize that children are not interested in your comfort or your sleep, while all you really care about is that they are good in both areas.

More times than you can begin to comprehend, this combo will leave you holding a sleeping baby in a chair, unwilling to move yourself or said baby for fear that their sleeping may end. You will be exhausted and want to catch a little shut-eye yourself, because you know, "Sleep when the baby sleeps" and all that.

But no one tells you that the baby will mostly be sleeping on you, and that you will mostly be sitting upright in a chair, so that sleeping when the baby sleeps will mean you battling gravity while trying to catch a few precious moments of shut-eye.

Sleeping while holding a baby is a lot like sleeping on an airplane, but without the booze and Dramamine to help you get comfortable. Just when you start to doze off while holding your baby, your head will flop forward, giving you whiplash. Or the side of your face will hit your shoulder, jarring you awake and leaving you with a black eye.

Practice this sleeping arrangement now and you will be handsomely rewarded with much-needed rest when the baby arrives. Personally, I was never able to pull off sleeping while sitting straight up, but I did get very good at sleeping with my head sideways, resting on my own shoulder. I'd wake up in terrible pain, because my neck was not a fan of being stretched to that degree, but the point is: I woke up. Which means I fell asleep. Which was worth a little neck pain.

The most important part of this exercise is for you to realize that you need a comfy nursery chair. Nursery room chair criteria should have padding and the ability to recline at the top of the list. When you are chair shopping aim more for that puffy La-Z-Boy recliner in your Uncle Larry's den and less for that adorable wooden rocking chair in the Pottery Barn catalog. Trust me; you won't give two shits how the chair looks in the nursery at 2 AM. And 3 AM. And 4 AM . . .

Partner Corner
BONDING WITH A BELLY

JEREMY: "I went to all the appointments I could for the first kid. Since it's not growing inside you, you are never gonna have the same connection a women does until it comes out. Once my boys came out, I loved them right away, no special bonding needed."

JASON: "I felt connected from the moment it happened, oddly enough. I know this is crazy, but I swear I knew from the moment it happened. I could not wait to meet my boys. I talked with them, played music, photographed the belly. Anything I could think of to make them know I cared about them."

BECKY: "I felt the babies kick. We bought a stethoscope and I tried listening to their heartbeats. I talked a lot to both of them. I went to all of Vivian's appointments, and I asked so many questions about what was happening and what was going to happen, just trying to understand it all."

MATT: "The first kid got the most in-utero singing/talking/ bad De Niro impressions. The subsequent younglings got belly rubs and good-night kisses. There is a lot of happiness in anticipation. Nine months is forever, then it's no time at all."

6

SOMETIMES
IT ALL GOES TO SHIT
Surviving a miscarriage

S O FAR WE'VE joked about most everything involved with
getting pregnant, being an embryonic host, and pushing
a watermelon out of your whooha. There are plenty of light
moments to discuss along the path of gestation, but no matter
how hard I try, I can't figure out a way to lighten up one thing
a lot of women have to endure in their journey to motherhood.

Miscarriage.

Because this book skews so sarcastic, I debated whether I
should even include a chapter on miscarriage. There is just
nothing funny or lighthearted to say about it. There is no witty
comment or bad joke that can help alleviate the effects of a miscarriage. And if sarcasm isn't an option, I'm not sure I'm of any
use to the conversation, really.

But it's estimated that 10 to 20 percent of known pregnancies end in miscarriage. That means that some of the pregnant
women reading this book are going to have their hearts broken
by miscarriage. Some women might be pregnant again, after suffering a miscarriage in the past. And all of the women reading are
probably scared shitless of having a miscarriage.

So even though I'm left to navigate this topic without my trusted brand of wit, I have still decided to push on. Because writing a book about pregnancy and not talking about miscarriage seems to be ignoring a very large, very sad elephant in the room.

Having no experience with miscarriage myself, I reached out to my MOFL to see if any of them had insight into the topic. In our tiny group, eight women had suffered a miscarriage. Eight. Several of them had suffered more than one.

I talked to four of these moms and I hope their stories can help you even a little tiny bit.

WHEN THE MISCARRIAGE HAPPENED

All of the moms I spoke to miscarried in their first trimester, most—but not all—before 10 weeks.

Amy was at her 12-week appointment when she learned she had miscarried, "I was having my first ultrasound and the female doctor was looking for the heartbeat. It was taking a while and I looked at my husband and said, 'I'm nervous.' The doctor replied, 'You should be. There's no heartbeat.' Pretty brutal way to find out."

Stephany had two miscarriages, one after a failed IVF, and the second when she miscarried one of her twins at 10 weeks. "With Logan's twin, we were completely blindsided at a doctor's appointment when his heartbeat was suddenly gone. We had already heard it several times, so it was tough. I had literally just gotten my head wrapped around having twins when it happened."

Corey miscarried three times, "I found out at my 12-week ultrasound that my twins both stopped at 6½ weeks. Then we found out at our 11-week ultrasound that the next baby stopped at 9 weeks. The third time I had slight cramping that kept increasing in pain. My spotting increased to full bleeding and I miscarried in about six hours."

Erika had a unique miscarriage, in that there was no bleeding involved: "I made an appointment because something just didn't feel right. The miscarriage was confirmed at the appointment. It was a 'missed miscarriage,' meaning that the baby had died, but my body didn't expel it, so it was not nearly as obvious as what normally happens. I had a tiny bit of spotting, but not enough to be concerned about generally speaking."

TELLING FRIENDS AND FAMILY

It's recommended that expectant parents wait until after the first trimester of pregnancy to announce that they have a baby on the way. This is because miscarriage is most common in the first trimester and it feels safer to hold off on announcing until those scary 12 weeks have passed.

This can be a really hard rule to follow when excited couples find out they are pregnant. They want to shout it from the rooftops (which sounds like a dangerous climb for a pregnant lady). A lot of people don't make it to the 12-week mark before they blurt it out to friends and family. I asked my MOFL if they waited to tell people about their pregnancies, and if they recommended waiting the 12 weeks, given their experiences.

Erika did the shouting from the rooftops the first time she found out she was pregnant: "I think when you are trying and then you get pregnant, you're insanely excited and want to tell the entire world. We did. It really sucked telling everyone the baby was lost afterward, but I don't think you could have kept me from telling people that first time. We were overjoyed and wanted to share our happiness."

After her miscarriage, she was much more reserved, "When we got pregnant the second time, we told no one. We weren't excited. We were terrified."

Amy thinks people should wait to tell everyone, because she wishes she had: "With the first pregnancy, we were so surprised and excited that we sent out a mass email announcing the news. I was probably eight weeks along. When I found out I had miscarried, I was embarrassed. I felt so stupid. I waited to tell anyone with the two pregnancies that I carried to term."

Stephany and her husband told her husband's parents early on with both of their miscarriages: "I kind of wish we wouldn't have. I felt like I had to comfort my mother-in-law because she was so upset for us. I would have preferred to just grieve in private."

While Stephany thinks people should wait to tell their friends and family, she also acknowledges that everyone is different, and it's a very personal choice when to announce a pregnancy: "Some people are super outgoing and share everything and rely on others for support." For people like that it makes sense to share their initial joy, even if it means having to share their sadness later.

THE EMOTIONAL EFFECT OF MISCARRIAGE

Miscarriage is an emotional wallop for all women, but my MOFL each processed theirs in a different way.

Erika stayed huddled up in a grief ball: "I didn't go to work for a week. I just stayed in bed and slept and cried. It was the worst heartbreak I've ever been through."

Amy also did quite a bit of crying: "I cried because I was so naive and didn't realize this happened to people. I cried because of loss. I cried because I had been so stupid to tell everyone so early. I cried because I felt I let people down. At some point I realized that it was really bad timing to get pregnant at that point in my life, and there was some relief. The relief made me feel guilty, so I cried. I was a fucking wreck."

Corey blamed herself for her losses: "I thought it was my fault. I was scared it would keep happening and that I would let my husband down in some way, since we always wanted more kids. I felt like I was letting my daughter down by not giving her siblings."

When Stephany miscarried she had already been through years of infertility and her mother's recent death. Her first miscarriage (a failed IVF) didn't hit her as hard as she expected it would: "I don't feel like my first miscarriage affected me tremendously. I was already emotionally drained and constantly verging on depression anyway. My thinking was, 'Well, at least I know I can get pregnant!' I thought we'd figure out a better IVF protocol and the next time would work for sure. I just tried to look at the positive."

Erika discovered that her miscarriage had lingering effects: "It kills the magic of finding out you're pregnant later. You're happy, but you're also fucking terrified that it will happen again. I remember when my husband and I found out about our first pregnancy. We were so happy we couldn't even speak. We were just hugging and laughing and crying. When we found out about the second pregnancy, it just wasn't the same. We agreed that if a second miscarriage happened, we wouldn't try again. It's just too much."

Amy was also very scared throughout the duration of her full-term pregnancy: "I never really celebrated the pregnancy like I wanted to because I just kept waiting for it to end."

I asked my MOFL if they had any advice for women who have gone through a miscarriage, and most of them came up pretty empty. I think they thought I was looking for some magic fix to pass on to other grieving moms, and none of them had anything magic to share.

Erika was not a huge fan of the comfort that was given to her following her miscarriage: "They tell you how common it is, and that it doesn't mean anything in terms of your general ability to have kids, but none of that really makes you feel any better. Your mind still spins off in horrible directions, and it's SO FUCKING HEARTBREAKING no matter what. I guess I would just say to give yourself time to grieve. It is real loss, and you have to let yourself process it on your own terms."

Amy came to appreciate some of the advice that she was given: "I hated hearing it at the time but I do believe everything happens for a reason. Whether it is because of a developmental abnormality or a chance to further solidify a relationship . . . I just feel like there is a reason it happens. I had so many miscarriages and it turned out to be because of a genetic mutation, where my body couldn't produce/convert folic acid and folate. Once my doctor found the cause, it took a year for me to get pregnant and keep the pregnancy going."

Stephany's infertility had taught her how to heal and move forward: "I think it's important to mourn in whatever way suits her and then move on. I know people who have fallen into a serious depression and can't even function after an early miscarriage. It's horrible and sad, but I guess it helped me not to dwell on it and to come up with our next game plan. However, our situation might be unique . . . or I may just be a heartless bitch! Who knows!"

While none of these women have a cure-all piece of advice for those who have had a miscarriage, it's worth noting that each of them kept trying to have kids. And each of them went on to give birth following their miscarriages. It's hard not to feel defeated when pregnancy ends, but it isn't defeat, it doesn't mark the end of your journey.

Amy has two healthy girls now, years after her first miscarriage: "I'm so appreciative of the health of my kids, because of all I endured. It just takes time to come to terms with it all."

So curl up in a ball, or call your best friend, or cry with your spouse, or make an appointment with your doctor to figure out what went wrong. Come to terms with your loss in whatever way feels right to you, so that you can heal in your own way and move forward when you are ready.

Partner Corner

Because a miscarriage happens to a woman's body, it can be difficult to remember that her partner suffers as well. A lot of times partners take it upon themselves to be a rock for their grieving spouse, leaving them little opportunity to process their own loss.

Corey's husband tried to take a logical approach to losing four babies, making the point that obviously the babies were not viable and miscarriage was a natural process. But she knows the losses hit him emotionally: "He still won't talk about them very much, so I think they affected him more than he is willing to let on. I know he didn't want me worrying about him."

Amy's husband was strong for her after their miscarriages. He did the heavy lifting of telling everyone the bad news following their first loss and took care of his grieving wife. But he wasn't letting on how sad he was as well: "About three weeks after it happened, we were in bed and I could feel the bed shaking. He was sobbing. I had no idea how sad he was and how much he was hurting too. It was really awful, but it brought us closer together. We started talking about it more and it was kind of our therapy."

Erika's husband tried to stay strong for her following their miscarriage, but finally cracked: "He was incredibly supportive and never cried until several days after. He broke down when I asked if he had told his family yet. The pain of actually telling them what happened let it all loose for him."

Stephany and her husband had their first miscarriage after years of infertility struggles. The ups and downs of trying to get pregnant had left Stephany rather numb, and it turns out her husband was the more emotional one: "He is very sweet and sensitive. I feel like he had the more stereotypical female response. He rushed home from work to be with me and he was so, so sad. I think he was surprised that I wasn't curled up on the floor sobbing or something. I just sort of moved on and was watching TV. Don't get me wrong; I was very sad. But I just didn't have the energy to be as sad as he was."

All of the women I spoke to said that they and their spouse reacted to their miscarriages differently. And each one said that forcing communication about the losses was an important part of moving forward together as a couple and into future pregnancies. Corey's advice is simple, yet perfect: "Talk to your partner even if the 'talking' is just crying or sitting silently together."

From the Partners

PETE: "Losing a child through a miscarriage is tough for dads too. The loss and vanquished expectations cut deep—and it caught me by surprise. I'm generally a stoic person and remain relatively unfazed by death, whether it's witnessing someone take their last breath (which, unfortunately has happened over a dozen times) or losing a close family member. But the miscarriage was different.

"There was an emptiness that I hadn't experienced before. Even more difficult was trying to figure out how to help my wife through it. I felt like I didn't have the right to grieve in the way she was. After all, I wasn't the one carrying the baby. It was my baby too, but I wasn't 'making' it like she was.

"It got even harder when we had to wait for her to pass the fetus. The job of recovering the fetus, bagging it, and preserving it to take to the doctor was the worst thing I have ever had to do—and I've done some difficult things when I was a police officer and fatal accident investigator. It haunted me for quite a while. Something I never told my wife—or anyone, until now.

"I knew I had to reassure her that the miscarriage wasn't her fault, but I didn't know how to do that or what to say. So I resorted to simply holding her, comforting her, and loving her. And in the end that worked."

JONATHAN: "It is sort of like a repressed memory—something I remember going through but all the feelings and pain have been replaced by the joy of having my healthy little girls.

I remember feeling extremely heartbroken, confused, frustrated, embarrassed. Even with all those things going on in my head, I think what really showed on the surface was the responsibility to help my wife through her side. I knew no matter how angry or sad I was, she was dealing with a whole different level of grief because it was happening inside of her. I needed to be the one to field phone calls and sympathy cards. I needed to be the one to appreciate kind words from friends and accept flowers. Thinking about it now, this job probably helped me cope because there was very little I could do to fix the problem.

"For a husband/partner dealing with this the first time I would just encourage them to support the other person. It isn't important why things are happening; it is just important to be there for each other. It isn't always going to be God's fault and it isn't always something that science can easily answer. Listen to what the other person is feeling and saying, even if you are feeling something different. Sometimes just being able to vent about concerns and frustrations in a safe way is therapeutic.

"Finally, time really does heal some of those wounds. It sounds super clichéd, but in the moment it feels like it's never going to get better. It always does. But I don't think it is something you can put a time stamp on or rush along."

WILL: "The next pregnancy was so frightful. At the first ultrasound, I nervously waited for that flicker on the screen showing a heartbeat. I kept thinking, 'Blink you little fucker, blink!' When he did, it was one of the happiest moments of my life."

Your Pregnancy Week by Week

HOW BIG IS YOUR BABY?

WEEK 8–JUNIOR MINT

Your baby is a little over ½ inch long this week. That is about the size of a Junior Mint. I think. I only eat Junior Mints in dark movie theaters, where I shovel them into my face by the handful, while hoping that the strangers sitting near me aren't judging.

WEEK 9–TATER TOT

At about 1 inch long, your baby is now the size of a Tater Tot. Tater Tots are deep-fried, which makes them better than any of the fruits and veggies that your pregnancy app compares your baby to.

WEEK 10–SUSHI YOU CAN'T EAT

Your baby is about the size of piece of a sushi roll, a little over 1 inch. You can't eat that sushi because it could hurt your baby, so maybe stop visualizing it.

2ND QUARTER
(11–20 weeks)

Your Pregnancy Week by Week
HOW BIG IS YOUR BABY?

WEEK 11—OREO COOKIE
Your baby is a little over 1½ inches long this week, which makes it about the size of an Oreo cookie. My pregnancy app said my baby was the size of a fig in week 11. I don't know what a fig is, other than when it's teamed up with a Newton in the cookie aisle. But even then, I've steered clear, because the word fig implies a level of healthy that sounds unacceptable for a cookie. So let's stick with Oreo.

WEEK 12—SHOT GLASS
Your baby is a little over 2 inches tall at this point, which makes him or her about the size of a shot glass. For many of you, this will remind you of the night your baby was conceived.

WEEK 13—CREAM CHEESE WONTON
There is a delicious appetizer they serve at some Chinese restaurants. They are little wontons filled with cream cheese, and they are about the size of your baby this week, 3 inches. If you haven't tried them before, you should, because (1) anything filled with cream cheese is delicious, and (2) once you have a child, your restaurant dining experience will not include such leisurely acts as ordering an appetizer.

WEEK 14—HANDFUL OF PRINGLES
At 3½ inches long, your baby is about the size of the average stack of Pringles I grab from the Pringles can for a snack. This is a very scientific example.

WEEK 15—TWINKIE
Your baby is 4 inches long this week, the same length as a Twinkie. You won't find Twinkies on most pregnancy apps, but you will find them deep-fried at fairs throughout the land, because this is the best country in the world.

Pregnancy WOD
MONTH 3

Now that you've spent a couple of months easing into your WOD, we are going to start throwing more difficult challenges your way. This month we are mixing physical and mental exercises.

Warning: Things are about the get messy. Proceed with caution.

1. Make an entire meal with one hand tied behind your back.

Once you have a baby, you will amaze yourself at the number of activities you will eventually be able to do using only one hand. You'll start to wonder why people even need two hands because you are kicking so much ass with only one. However, the learning curve to the kicking of ass can be a steep one, so you might as well start climbing it now.

Tie your hand behind your back, or hold Baby Flour on your hip as you go about your normal daily routine. Even if your normal daily routine doesn't involve cooking in the kitchen, go ahead and practice on that skill anyway. There's an off-chance you might not be able to eat every meal at a restaurant once you have a child. Figure out how that oven and stove of yours works, and maybe even chop up a vegetable or two.

Yes, you'll probably slice off at least part of your finger, and you might even accidently catch Baby Flour on a little bit of fire. But that is what these exercises are for; the goal is to avoid blood and bodily harm once your real child arrives. So get all of your cooking-related ER trips out of the way in advance.

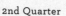

2. Have an entire argument with your spouse where each of you is not allowed to talk above a whisper.

Even the best relationships will be put the test in the first months (years?) of parenthood. Sleep deprivation and general parenting incompetence can combine for some rather heated exchanges in the early days. Often these exchanges take place in the middle of the night and within earshot of the baby.

Not wanting to expose an alert baby to parental squabbles, or to wake a sleeping baby, parents will be forced to have most of their arguments in nothing louder than a whisper. It can be difficult to get used to whispering obscenities, but if you start now you'll be a pro by the time you have a child audience to your marital dysfunction.

3. Sprint around the grocery store, filling up your cart with necessary items. Abandon said cart just before you get to the checkout counter. Flee to your car.

Do you remember that game show from the '90s called *Supermarket Sweep*? Oh my goodness, did I love that show. The main point of the show was for people to run around a store and fill their grocery carts with as much food as they could in a set amount of time. There was screaming, throwing of expensive cheese, and very questionable fashion choices involving a lot of sweaters.

If you don't remember that show, you should probably take a moment to Google a clip. Study that clip of chaos and flying food and absorb it. Because that is what you are going to look like once you start shopping with a child in tow. The only difference is that your fashion choices will most likely be even more unfortunate.

No longer will you have the luxury of meandering through aisles, grabbing items as you remember needing them. Once you have a baby, meandering is off the menu, as is your memory.

So you'll need to make a list, then you'll need to move with the speed of the fastest Supermarket Sweeper that ever swept. Because you are not in charge of this trip; your baby is. At any moment, your sleeping or cooing baby can decide your time has run out and you are officially eliminated from the competition. At that point you will be forced to abandon your cart, no matter how full it is, and quickly exit the store. Maybe you'll have better luck next time. (But odds are you won't be dressed any better, let's be honest.)

Getting prepared for this new way of shopping is a great use of your pregnancy time. Learn every item in every aisle of your store. Devise the quickest route for covering all the aisles you will need. Locate the bathrooms for the diaper explosions that inevitably happen during every trip. Practice abandoning your cart and fleeing from the store with only a few seconds notice. And get the supermarket staff used to seeing you in sweatpants and no makeup, as that will be your shopping attire from here on out.

Ready, go!

YOU HAVE 99 EMOTIONS, AND YOU'RE GOING TO HIT EVERY ONE

Bystanders beware

7

$\mathscr{I}$'M NOT BIG on emotions. If you were to make a chart of my emotions, you'd end up with pretty much a straight line down the middle: not too happy, not too sad. Except for the occasional spike of road rage or losing my patience with an incompetent help line operator, I've never spent too much time wading outside of my pretty reserved emotional waters.

Until I got pregnant.

And ooo-whee, did that chart start adding some peaks and valleys.

Not every woman will notice a big change in her emotions when she gets pregnant, but for those of us who do notice, it comes as a bit of a shock to our very calm systems.

At one of my doctor's appointments I found out that I had a urinary tract infection that was going to require antibiotics to clear up. My doctor told me that it could have been caused by not drinking enough water. I lost my mind and started hysterically crying. *Hysterically.*

I don't cry. Hysterically or otherwise.

I didn't want to take any medicine, because I was convinced it would hurt the baby. But the doctor said that the infection could spread and that would definitely hurt the baby.

I cried all the way home. I called my mom and cried as I drove. When I got home I walked into Becky's office, still hysterically crying. She was on the phone. She immediately hung up because she thought something horrible had happened.

I put the antibiotics on her desk and said it was all my fault, that I hadn't drunk enough water, that I was a terrible mother, and the baby was going to be hurt because of it. Becky still wasn't sure what the hell was going on. I had now moved into the hiccup, gasping-for-breath part of the crying, so she couldn't actually understand what I was saying.

The crying continued for quite some time. Becky had never seen me cry, and now I had snot pouring out of my nose because I was in hysterics. And she was in shock.

A similar situation unraveled late one evening when our cat brought a nearly dead bird home to share. I sat on the stairs in the backyard while the bird died and I cried as if my cat had just slaughtered my best friend before my eyes. Even more snot pouring from my face.

My crying fits were just part of my new emotional repertoire. I also had flashes of anger, confusion, impatience, anxiety, and manic happiness. I was just a ball of fun.

Becky and I both understood that these emotions were obviously a result of my pregnancy, but that didn't automatically make them easier to deal with. Neither of us was used to my being so moody, and it was hard to adjust to my sudden onset of hysterics.

If you are struggling to navigate your newly choppy emotional waters, all I can say is have patience with yourself. Take a lot of deep breaths, try to talk yourself down when you are about to go over a crazy cliff, and if you end up on the other side of the cliff, try to apologize to those you may have taken out along the way. Nobody will fault a pregnant lady for going a little batty, but it never hurts to acknowledge the batty after you've had some time to calm down a bit.

And look at it this way, this range of emotions is nothing compared to what is coming your way once you add a baby and sleep deprivation to your schedule. So just think of this time as dress rehearsal for the real show that is about to start.

Moms on the Front Lines

A MESS OF EMOTIONS

SARAH: "I cried in Build-A-Bear when I was pregnant and Drew was giving up his pacifier by putting it in a bear. My poor dad was there and he didn't know what to do with me!"

TARA: "I was more emotional postpartum with my first pregnancy. The second time around, it was worse during pregnancy. My son finally got used to seeing me cry. At first it really bothered him. Eventually he just rolled his eyes and was like, 'Is she ever going to stop?'"

ERIKA: "I lost what little sense of direction I had when I was trying to meet my husband for lunch one day. The place was walking distance and I'd been there several times, but I could not figure out how to get there, even with the assistance of Google Maps. By the time my husband finally located me, I was absolutely hysterical. Talk about losing your shit. The bizarre thing was that I was keenly aware of how ridiculous I was being, but could not for the life of me stop and get it together."

Partner Corner

SHE'S CRAZY

Partners, if I teach you only one thing in the course of this book, let this be it. Never, I mean never, point out to a pregnant lady that she is being overly emotional. Just don't. Don't try to rationalize with her by explaining that her pregnancy is causing her mood swings. Another don't.

Even if she says something like, "This pregnancy is making me so crazy!" This is a trap; do not fall into it. Do not agree with that statement, because, as she just pointed out, she is not of sound mind. And if you agree with her, all she will hear is you calling her crazy. Don't let her hear that.

The proper response is, "Aw, no it's not; you're doing great! Do you want some ice cream or a foot rub?" Always err on the side of offering treats and relaxation. Remember this survival tip forever.

Also, I have some not-great news for you. Your Baby Mama's emotions aren't going to magically self-correct as soon as the child pops out. So don't go expecting that. Once the baby arrives, she'll be battling postpartum blues and exhaustion. And even after that, she'll forever be carrying the weight of parenthood around at all times, so she may never be fully returned to her former relaxed glory.

But don't point that out. Ever. Just go with your trusty standby, "You're doing great! Do you want some ice cream or a foot rub?" Always go with that.

From the Partners

BECKY: "I thought I was pretty good about letting my partner run with these new emotions. They didn't make sense to either of us so I tried to just support her through them."

JASON: "On the emotional roller coaster that was her second pregnancy, I was just there to support her and talk her through tough emotional states or just give her a hug."

KEVIN: "I was pretty practical about it. You have to keep your head on, because someone has to be able to process things in a consistent, actionable manner, or you'll go crazy thinking about the weight of what's going on. I just made my mind up to do whatever I could do to make my wife as comfortable as possible."

Pregnancy WOD
MONTH 4

A lot of people wait until the three-month mark to announce their pregnancy, making month four the first month that you might start to feel like this whole thing is actually real. In the spirit of keeping it real, we are going to start ramping things up this month. It's time to get serious about this.

1. Eat a meal with one hand tied behind your back.

This task comes after you've perfected cooking with one hand, because you are going to need the skills required to actually eat your meal with only one hand as well. Eating while holding a baby is a unique balancing exercise, in that you are trying very hard to get your face close enough to your plate to catch some food, and are also required to keep your baby as far away from the plate as possible, because he or she wants nothing more than to throw your food across the room. It's an attractive balance, to be sure.

Grab your handy bag of flour and sit down for your meal. Do not sit down like a normal person would—instead, sit down almost perpendicular to your plate, with your dominant hand nearest the table and your flour situated as far away from the table as you can manage without dropping it on the kitchen floor.

Now, eat. Do not take your time, do not dilly-dally. The point of the meal is to get sustenance into your body as quickly as possible, because at any point your bag of flour may decide this dinner party is over. Your bag will decide this by crying, pooping, spitting up, or managing to grab your plate of food and throw it

THE SH!T NO ONE TELLS YOU

to the ground in protest of there being even a single moment not dedicated exclusively to its needs.

Put your face down near the plate and shovel food into it with abandon. It's okay if some misses; just keep moving forward. Hopefully you have a dog or Roomba to assist with mealtime cleanup (if not, this would be an excellent time to get both). Buy yourself a little shoveling time by bouncing the flour on your knee while you eat. If there is something that needs to be cut on your plate, you should probably just pick it up with your hands and rip it apart with your teeth, because getting a knife involved in this unsteady setup could lead to disaster.

Once you've mastered leaning into the table while holding the baby away from the table, there is one more advanced move you can practice if you are feeling ambitious. Grab a baby bottle with your flour-holding hand, and feed it to the bouncing bag while you eat your food. I warn you that this combination is not for amateurs and can often lead to your bouncing your fork into your eye because you messed up your rhythm. Sharp utensils are not recommended.

2. Get up at 2 AM, strip, and completely remake a bed in your house. Without making any noise.

Before you have kids you don't have much occasion to jump out of bed and into immediate action in the middle of the night. Unless you have cats and you hear them hacking up a fur ball or bringing in a half-dead bird to share with you at 1 AM (aren't cats a delight?).

Babies will cry and need you at random times throughout the night for months and years. You'll get so quick at reacting that you'll find yourself sitting in their nursery, boob out to breast-feed, even when it's just the hacking cat that woke you up. But it's still important that you get used to the unique feeling of panic, chaos, and disorientation that comes with being startled awake and made to function within seconds.

So set a blaring alarm on your phone and pop out of bed the second you hear the alarm. Run down the hallway and strip the bed in your spare room. Then rummage through the storage closets to find replacement bedding. Remake the bed. Do all this in the dark, without making any noise.

If you and your partner do this fire drill a few times a week until the baby comes, your hearts and your minds will be well equipped for the late-night antics of your tiny offspring.

3. Go to Chuck E. Cheese on a Friday night and stay for 1½ hours. Touch at least four different game surfaces.

This month we are developing our tolerance not only for noise, but also germs. Children bring along an immeasurable amount of both. If you can survive a few visits to Chuck E. Cheese without losing your mind or ending up with an incurable illness you are well prepared for parenting.

4. While at Chuck E. Cheese, strike up conversations with complete strangers. Make plans to hang out and have coffee with them and their children at a later date.

Remember how fun it was to go to bars and make small talk with random people in the hope of them becoming a sex partner of yours? Don't you miss the awkwardness of those exchanges, the uncertainty you felt when meeting someone new, and the wonders it all did for your self-esteem?

I have good news for you! You are about to enter into another era of small talk and awkwardness! This era is called the Time of Socializing with Any Parent Who Has a Kid the Same Age as Yours!

Just when you thought you were done having to impress strangers in social settings, you went and decided to have a kid. And you will probably decide to socialize that kid. You see where this is heading.

This time, you won't be meeting strangers in dark bars with booze in your hand. Instead your encounters will now take place in bright rooms full of children and noise. Caffeine will be the strongest drug present, but its presence will be required for survival of all adults in attendance.

Now, of course, there are ways to avoid interacting with other moms, and to remain steadfast in your desire to never engage in small talk again. You can fiddle with your phone during kid activities and parties. You can stay quiet and withdrawn in social situations. And I'll admit that I've done all of the above on days when the thought of exerting one more ounce of energy was too much for my brain to bear.

But on the whole, it's usually worth striking up a conversation with parents who have kids the same age as yours. They understand where you are coming from, without much explanation required. They sympathize with your struggles and often can help you through them. And more than anything, there is the chance that your kid can be entertained by their kid, leaving you the chance to have a conversation with a person who isn't simultaneously soiling themselves while you chat. You have no idea how exciting that will sound after you have a baby.

So dust off those socializing skills and work on a few mom-friendly pickup lines, because it won't be long until you are back in the game.

THE SH!T NO ONE TELLS YOU

Dear Bean Letters
Week 19, Sick

Dear Bean,

I've been pregnant for a while now. I'm excited and nervous and more than a little clueless. But most of all I'm nauseous. All the time. There's a feeling people get just before they are going to puke; I have that feeling 24 hours a day, but have managed to avoid the actual puking so far. The all-day nausea has helped take my mind off of being nervous and clueless, so at least I have that going for me.

I'm sure most expectant moms spend their time Googling a myriad of questions about pregnancy, babies, and parenting. I've dabbled a bit in those subjects from time to time, but at least once a day I ask the dear internets, "How long does morning sickness last?"

I'm not sure why I ask so often, and I'm not sure whether I think that Google will somehow alert my stomach that it's time to stop it with the torture.

Google has told me every day for weeks that morning sickness is supposed to ease up around week 13 or 14 of pregnancies. Before I reached week 13 or 14, I would wake up every morning and open the pregnancy app on my phone, literally counting down the days to week 13. Because week 13 was going to bring relief! Google demanded it!

I'm in week 19 now and my body has given a big middle finger to Google and its "facts." Not only is my morning sickness not just contained to the morning hours, it is also extending past the magic 13-week cut-off time. It's an overachiever, this sickness.

The good news is I'm the only pregnant person I know that has found my first couple of trimesters to be an excellent weight-loss regimen. I've lost 10 pounds since getting pregnant, because it turns out that feeling like you are going to puke 24 hours a day doesn't inspire a lot of snacking.

My doctor has mentioned that if I start puking, they may have to put me on some anti-nausea medication, because then I would be puking up what little nutrients I'm managing to get in my belly. Recently a report came out about the anti-nausea medication they gave pregnant women 30 years ago. The report was not positive, and the effects on the babies was even less so. So I am doing all I can to avoid the puking and any anti-nausea medicine.

I've been eating a lot of crackers and having a lot of heart-to-hearts with my stomach about the need to hold on to what little food I manage to eat. I do not want to take any medication, and the only way to avoid that is to get enough food into my belly to keep the both of us healthy. Here's hoping that toast is enough to build an entire person from scratch. I put butter on it, to really make it a complete meal.

Mama, in an attempt to be helpful, constantly asks me what I want to eat, as if getting me what I want will somehow make eating more enjoyable. I constantly answer, "Nothing. I don't want to eat anything. Make me something, put it in front of me, and I will do intense breathing exercises to force it into my belly."

So you can see, it's been a real special time for the both of us.

There is an old wives' tale that babies with dark hair give their moms worse morning sickness than other babies. It's also said that girls make their moms sicker than boy babies. We already know you are a girl. And apparently you might be a monkey, covered from head to toe in dark hair.

People, including my doctors, have told me that morning sickness is a sign of a really healthy pregnancy. I'm 95 percent sure this is complete crap fabricated to make me feel better about feeling horrible for five months. "It just took me 10 minutes to chew and swallow a piece of toast, because every part of my being wants to expel it from my body. But that just means the baby is really, really healthy! I'm so lucky!"

Complete crap.

But here's the thing. I've been so, so scared of losing you, from the second I found out I was pregnant. At only six weeks pregnant, I felt a little cramping and rushed to the doctor. I cried when they said it was too early to confirm anything on an ultrasound. They told me my blood tests seemed fine, that I seemed fine, that everything was probably fine.

I didn't believe them. I continued to worry.

Every time I've gone into one of my appointments I've held my breath while they searched for your little galloping heartbeat. Each time part of me expects it not to be there, for this dream to all come crashing down. It's all so theoretical, this pregnancy, you, what is happening inside of me.

But that's why this morning (really all-day) sickness comes in handy. Although I don't believe this nausea is proof that I have a

➤

healthy baby, it is a reminder that, yes, something real is happening inside me. If I wasn't growing a baby, I wouldn't feel like shit 24 hours a day. If I wasn't still pregnant, I might actually perk up at the thought of a meal.

I can't feel you moving yet, and until I can, I will constantly be wondering whether you are okay. But until then, as I sit here at the dining room table with my head in my hands, taking deep breaths between every bite, I smile a little. Because this is your way of letting me know you're still swimming in there.

Or that you are a monkey.

Could go either way.

8

MOMMY WARS
START NOW

You best come prepared with your A-game

Have you heard of the Mommy Wars? They are the real or imagined competitions among moms over who is the best parent. Are the stay-at-home moms providing a better life for their offspring than the working moms? Are the Pinterest moms crafting their way to happy childhoods for their kids? If your child isn't enrolled in 13 extracurricular activities by the age of nine months, will they inevitably end up in prison or on a stripper pole? Are you failing spectacularly at mommyhood, while Cheryl down the street seems to have it all put together (and she made it all from scratch)?

I say the Mommy Wars are both real and imagined, because there really are moms out there who seem to always be in competition mode and who never fail to judge others who aren't performing as well. But in reality, I think there are probably more of us judging ourselves than there are moms sitting around giving two shits about whether other people's kids are eating organic. I mean, Cheryl doesn't have time for that, she has a new slow cooker recipe to make.

But whether or not Mommy Wars are actually real, they feel real. And the place where they feel the most real is on social media. Social media is where the Mommy Wars have really taken off, because the Internet offers a unique space where everyone can share only the positive parts of their lives. And even though we all know we are only posting the positive parts of our lives, we still find it difficult to do the math and realize that Cheryl is doing the same thing.

So we look at Cheryl's posts and think, "Look at how great her life is! I bet it's like that all day every day, even though a photo is literally a split second in time." Then we feel bad because obviously Cheryl has her shit together in a way we just never will.

In addition to Cheryl's family perfection, she also shares articles about all the different things parents should be doing to ensure they are not raising a serial killer. Cheryl posts a lot of articles, because apparently there are a lot of different ways children can turn into serial killers. We don't have time to read all of the articles, let alone implement the anti–serial-killer habits, so Cheryl has once again left us feeling defeated.

As a newbie to this mommy world, you might not realize until it's too late that you are participating in the Mommy Wars. You've mostly ignored Cheryl's posts over the years, because you didn't have kids and have had no need to make American Girl Doll clothes by hand. The parenting articles Cheryl posted didn't have anything to do with reality TV or travel destinations, so you scrolled right past them.

But then you got pregnant.

And then you were officially drafted into the Mommy Wars, whether you liked it or not. Whether you knew it or not. All of a sudden, Cheryl's articles start stressing you out. And her meal planning and craft playdates and beautifully coordinated children seem like more than you can manage.

Maybe you expected to be given a reprieve from competition until your actual child arrived. How innocent you were.

The only way to survive the Mommy Wars is to be on the top of your game from day one. As soon as social media knows that you are harboring a human child in your uterus, it will move swiftly to provide its opinion on all things fetus, pregnant lady, and anti–serial-killer parenting techniques. You need to be on point and immediately let social media know that you intend to be a fierce competitor in this completely fabricated game that means nothing in the scheme of things.

Game face on, ladies!

PREGNANCY ANNOUNCEMENT

This is where it all starts. If you don't come out of the gate strong, you may never catch up. Hopefully you started planning this announcement well before you even got pregnant, because that's what winners do, and if you are going to win at parenting, you had better be putting in the hours it takes to succeed.

If you are an amateur, it will be hard for you to gauge the success of your pregnancy announcement. You may get excited and think you did a good job simply because your post gets a lot of likes. But this is one of the few posts where "likes" mean very little in calculating its potency.

I mean, you are announcing that your body is in the beginning process of making a human child. Everyone is going to throw a like your way for that. Even a simple "I'm preggers!" post would get more likes than pretty much anything you've ever posted. But if you are only bringing an "I'm preggers!" post to this game, you are setting yourself up for defeat.

These days, if your announcement doesn't go viral, then you are a complete failure at parenting before you've even started parenting. It's really that simple. We are going to need to see some real orchestration involved in this announcement. If you are only going to post a photo, that photo better be a professional one. It better involve props and a play on words and inspire your friends and family to hit that "Share" button with abandon.

But to be honest, photos are so five years ago.

If you really want to compete in the pregnancy announcement game, you are going to need to move up to moving pictures. We've all seen the countless pregnancy announcement videos and we've all oohed and aahed and cried along with them. Your pregnancy announcement needs to make people openly weep if it has any hope of success.

Pregnancy Announcement Scoring

This handing scoring guide will help you push yourself and your announcement to the next level. If your planned announcement adds up to fewer than 30 points, go back to the drawing board, because this is the future of your child we are talking about.

- Ultrasound Image—10 points
- Props—10 points
- Cheesy jokes or puns—5 points
- Video reveal of your pregnancy to your partner, parent, or close friend—10 points
- Video of your partner, parent, or close friend crying with joy at the reveal—15 points
- Video of your partner, parent, or close friend letting out a slew of f-bombs at the reveal—25 points
- Singing—15 points
- Choreography—10 points
- Humor—10 points
- Tears—10 points
- Jumping—10 points

GENDER ANNOUNCEMENT

When I announced my first baby on social media, I posted an ultrasound image and said something to the effect of, "I can't wait to meet her!" And that was the extent of my announcement about my pregnancy and the gender of my child. There's a possibility I might be kicked off social media if I put that little effort into a gender announcement these days.

If you are finding out the gender of your baby before it is born, it is now mandated by law that you do so in a completely over-the-top way. There needs to be a party. There need to be props. There need to be baked goods with pink or blue filling. I don't make up the rules; I just report them.

Your baby's gender announcement will probably involve even more planning than the Pregnancy Announcement. As you've probably noticed all over social media, these announcements have taken on a life of their own. Is that a wedding video you are watching? No, it is not. That is a video of a gender-reveal party. It looks like a wedding because there are 100 people in attendance, 300 balloons, flowers, appetizers, sign-in books, and cake. Always cake.

Since I generally take a pro-cake stance in all areas of life (it's important to have principles), I don't really have a problem with a gender-reveal party. And throwing a big party to announce the gender of your unborn baby is an excellent way to let it be known that you aren't messing around when it comes to this mommy game.

But if you really want to make your mark, you are going to need to think outside of the pink or blue cake idea. Maybe open a big box of pink or blue balloons that fly up into the air while your crowd cheers. Maybe hit a piñata full of pink or blue confetti. Or have people throw confetti on you. Or have friends pellet you with water guns full of pink or blue paint. But probably don't explode anything causing pink or blue smoke, because people have done that and the police didn't think it was a great idea. Are these police aware of the Over-the-Top Gender-Reveal Mandate that is in effect? Apparently not.

PREGNANCY ACCOMPLISHMENTS

Even though you are quite busy building a person and a placenta inside of your body, it is crucial to remember that there are still important things to attend to outside of your uterus. Most worthy of your attention are the annoying pregnant women running wild on social media accomplishing all sorts of ridiculous things despite the fact that building a placenta gives you an automatic free pass to sit on the couch and eat ice cream for nine months.

These overachievers are completing half marathons at five months pregnant, doing CrossFit up until their due dates, and assembling a nursery that looks like the "After" photos on one of those home makeover shows you watch while sitting on the couch eating ice cream.

Their ambition and energy is making you look bad, and frankly it's quite annoying.

These women mark the true beginning of your introduction to the Mommy Wars, because the feeling you get when you look at their overly ambitious pregnancy posts is very similar to the feeling you are going to get after your kid arrives and you have to constantly see Cheryl posting about how much parenting ass she is kicking.

There's not really much you can do to battle the ambitious pregnant women. There's no party you can throw or video you can post to compete with their athleticism and overall can-do attitude. I mean, it's not like you are all of a sudden going to take up long-distance running at 20 weeks pregnant (seriously, don't do that). And your binge watching every episode of *The Wire* is probably not quite the same as their challenging themselves to do 30 burpees a day in their third trimester (although *The Wire* does deal with some really complex themes, so it's almost the same).

But that's not to say you don't have options. One of my favorite responses to social media perfectionism is to post the most unperfect image of my life that I can find. Your pregnant friend posted a picture of herself at the finish line of her latest run? Counter that with a picture of your cankles. Her nursery design is featured in *Perfect Mothers Monthly*? Your nursery is just a pile of gift bags and one old rocker your mom bought at a garage sale. Post it. She's "barely showing" at 30 weeks? You are constantly asked if you are having triplets at 23 weeks. Post it.

Develop your mommy sarcasm early and it will serve you well as you wade deeper and deeper into these battlefields. And you know what you can do while developing sarcasm? Eat ice cream on the couch. Win, win.

NEWBORN PHOTOS

No matter what you have done throughout your pregnancy, no matter how well you have competed in the Mommy Wars thus far, you will be awarded zero points if you do not have adorable newborn photos to share with the masses. Do not falter here, ladies.

Because adorable is an absolute requirement, your Official Newborn Photo cannot be one that you have taken yourself. See, it turns out newborns aren't actually that cute, and your phone isn't actually that great of a camera. This is a dangerous combination and should not be trusted during such an important time.

Start researching newborn photographers well before your due date. Look through their portfolio, confirm that they are able to make newborn babies look adorable (spoiler alert: they have some excellent editing software that greatly assists in this effort). Find a photographer that will come to your house and has reasonable rates (make sure you get all your digital files included in their fee) and lock them down.

As soon as you have the baby, let the photographer know and get them out for a shoot within the first week or so. No, you won't feel like being photographed in the first week, but get over it. Babies do a lot of sleeping that first week or so, which means they are a lot easier to photograph and pose in buckets and on baseball gloves or whatever other contortions you come up with.

You need to get in the photos as well, even though you look and feel like crap. Throw on some makeup and ask your sweet photographer to use her editing software to make you look better than Cheryl, please.

You might not want to spend the money on a professional photographer. Or you might feel too overwhelmed in those first couple of weeks to let anyone into your house, let alone someone who is there to document what is happening. But the Mommy

Wars are not for the squeamish, or for those without editing software at their disposal.

This is your child's introduction to social media, an unveiling of sorts. You have come this far, suffered through cankles and contractions; do not shy away from this big moment.

Hire the professional, throw the baby in a bucket, put four gallons of concealer on your face, and get out there to compete!

We are coming for you, Cheryl.

Moms on the Front Lines

MOMMY WARS

MONICA: "I hear about it all the time but I think I naturally distance myself from anyone like this so I don't feel many effects. But I have friends who talk about it. I have zero time or energy to invest in this."

MICHELLE: "When I had my first baby I definitely felt the Mommy Wars. I knew a few moms who were constantly preaching the rights and wrongs of mommyhood. They always seemed like their life was perfect. I felt extremely inadequate as a first-time mom as a result of Mommy Wars. Over the years, I have distanced myself from those few moms and surrounded myself with an awesome village of women who don't feel the need to compete. Instead, these women are always willing to lend an extra hand, help out with carpool, keep an eye on the kids, give heartfelt advice, and most important, reassure one another that we are all doing the best we can."

Partner Corner

JEREMY: "All the dads I know think that the 'mom competitions' are dumb. Our competing is done in high school, sometimes college. More of how fast your car is, how pretty your girlfriend is, how much you can drink. I don't feel competitive toward the dudes that are my friends or that I associate with. Dudes are just there to enjoy the company and bullshit and help one another out. And complain about shit."

Pregnancy WOD
MONTH 5

You are officially halfway through your pregnancy. You may have found out the gender of your baby at your 20-week appointment and have now started shopping for blue or pink with abandon. While it is okay to enjoy this time, please do not lose focus on your ultimate goal: surviving your newborn baby. Blue and pink will do nothing to save you, but your Pregnancy WODs will. So stay diligent, continue to get your parenthood muscles in shape, and you will be fully prepared for that little blue or pink ball of dynamite that is coming your way. Go, team!

1. Throw a pen, a carrot, a hand towel, a bottle nipple, and bag of M&M's on the floor. Pick each item up with your toes.

The only real skill I've developed over the course of my years as a parent is the ability to pick up just about anything off the floor with my toes. When I first brought my babies home, I was too sore to bend over and pick stuff up; then they got heavier and I was too out of shape to bend or squat down while holding them (well, the squatting wasn't difficult; it was getting back up from the squat that proved impossible). After years of picking stuff up with my feet, I got so damn good at it I started to rely primarily on my toes for grabbing things, just because I could.

I have even added a little flip at the end of the pickup, where I toss the item in the air with my feet and catch it with my hand. Obviously, you are not at that level yet. And I don't want you beating yourself up if you struggle with these beginner skills, while

I've moved on to a competitive level. Keep your focus and you too can one day throw a baby carrot in the air with your feet and catch it with your hands. We are making dreams come true here.

2. Have a drunk person set four alarms on your phone to go off at random times during the night.

When the alarms go off, run into another room of your house and comfort your bag of flour for 30 minutes before going back to bed. Also, maybe just have the drunk person stay over and deal with them throughout the night. Their puking, bladder control issues, unexplained crying, and general inability to communicate coherently will be great practice for a baby.

3. Locate a cat. Strap that cat into a car seat in the back of your car. Go for an hour-long drive on the freeway.

Driving with a new baby can be an audio and psychological torture unlike anything you've ever experienced. Your baby is new to this world, only wants to be close to you, and for some reason has been abandoned after being strapped down into a holding device. Your baby will not understand this chain of events and more to the point, will not tolerate it.

There will be screaming and crying, first from the baby, and gradually from the parent who is driving as well. You will try to calm your baby with soothing promises, but your baby won't hear any of that shit because you have clearly left them to perish in the backseat of a car while you are off doing God only knows what. They will scream louder, hoping maybe a kind stranger will take pity and save them.

The fact that babies scream is not something that should take you by surprise, but there is something uniquely awful about hearing your baby scream just beyond your reach, with no way for you to comfort them. It goes against every instinct in your soul, and it slowly breaks that soul over the course of a drive.

So grab a cat and strap it in the backseat. Cats do not enjoy cars or being strapped down, and will most likely wail in a way that is similar to that of your upcoming child. Head out on the freeway for a drive. Freeways are unique in their torture because they do not offer the opportunity to pull over and comfort the cat. Also, freeways require extra attention be paid to driving, because of the high speeds. This means it's not safe to reach back and try to comfort the cat with a gentle touch (and cats aren't big on being gently touched when they are freaking the hell out, so probably don't even bother trying that one).

Your cat, just like your baby, will have no idea what you are saying when you are trying to soothe it, so it will help you get used to being completely useless in this scenario.

If you do this exercise more than once, you are going to need to find a new cat each time. There will be blood (yours) if you try to wrangle a cat into your car more than once. (Save that exercise for your Toddler WOD).

4. Before leaving the house, grab approximately 18 items into your hands and take them with you to the car. The combined weight of the items must be at least 35 pounds. Don't forget to grab your flour, too.

Babies themselves aren't really that big. But you will soon discover that babies do not travel without an entourage. A heavy and cumbersome entourage. Pre-baby, you can decide to leave the house, and then a mere seconds later, you can actually walk out of said house. It's a very exciting time in your life, to be sure.

These good ol' days will come to screeching halt the first time you try to leave the house with a baby in tow. Sure, theoretically you could just grab the baby and the car seat and be on your way. But once you are out of the house with only a baby and a car seat, it will become painfully obvious that you are unable to parent without the help of quite a few accessories.

You'll need a diaper bag full of diapers, butt creams, wipes, bottles, bibs, backup clothes, burp cloths, binkies, back-up clothes to the back-up clothes, nursing covers, toys, and roughly 382 additional items that basically make you a mobile Babies "R" Us store. You'll also need blankets, and maybe a stroller, a travel Boppy is nice, a Bjorn might come in handy, and anything else that may help keep either you or the baby sane for the duration of your adventure into society.

Prepare yourself for your upcoming exit struggles by running around the house and gathering up 18 items every time you are about to leave. Pile them all into your arms and only make one trip to the car, because making more than one trip is for sissies.

Use these pregnancy months to build up your arm muscles, your speed, and your balance while carrying 35 pounds worth of items to and from your car. Your neighbors may be confused, but don't let their judgmental stares slow you down.

9

PINK, BLUE, OR YELLOW
To gender or not to gender

$\mathcal{Y}$OU WILL FIND that once you are to the showing stage of your pregnancy (when people can actually tell you are pregnant, and not just bloated from a visit to a large buffet), you will constantly be asked if you know what gender you are having. Then you will be asked if you are excited or disappointed about that gender, as if that is an appropriate question to ask a person. If you happen to say that you aren't finding out the gender, you will be met with looks of confusion and fear. Which, again, is totally appropriate.

Deciding whether to find out the gender of your baby in advance is an extremely personal choice and one that you probably made long before you even got pregnant. Because you've known for a long time what kind of person you are.

If you are like me, you know full well that there is no way on God's green earth that you would be able to wait 40 weeks to find out the gender of your child. So it probably never even crossed your mind. What did cross your mind was to stock up on those over-the-counter gender-reveal pee tests that you can take as early as 10 weeks along. Because, as with me, patience is probably not one of your stronger qualities.

For those of you who were blessed with a weaker Control Freak gene, you may be excited to wait until your child arrives to find out their gender. This will be the biggest surprise of your life and you can wait a few extra months to make the reveal all that more fun. While I have a lot of respect for your willpower, I have some questions about your logic.

I've never really understood the "There are only so many good surprises in life, why not wait to find out?" argument. I mean, how surprised are you really going to be? You are birthing a child, a human child. That much is known. This isn't the *Price Is Right*. It's not like you are going to push and then they are going to hold up a big-screen TV or maybe a trip to Italy and say, "Surprise! Look what you have won!" Spoiler alert: It's going to be a child. It's going to have one of two possible genital situations happening. It's not *that* surprising.

And isn't it equally surprising to find out at week 12 as it is to find out after 40 weeks and 26 hours of labor? After screaming and drugs and pushing and cussing and kicking a nurse do you really care if it's a boy or a girl? No, you are just happy to have it out of you, no matter its genitalia.

The only people who get a *real* surprise in regard to gender are the ones who are told the wrong sex by their ultrasound technician. The ones who vomit pink all over their baby's nursery and then push a penised child out at their delivery. This scenario was always in the back of my mind as I got closer to my due date, and each time we had a backup name picked just in case a different gender popped out.

Since we chose half of our children's DNA from a sperm bank, I also always wondered whether the guy we chose from the binder was actually the sperm we received. I mean, there was no way to know for sure if it had been switched; it's not like the vials had distinguishing features. I joked throughout the pregnancy that our baby could pop out and be an unexpected race. Now *that* would be a fun surprise. Much more exciting than the big-screen TV.

Moms on the Front Lines
TO WAIT OR REVEAL

AMY: "I waited to find out with both, which was shocking, seeing as how I'm super OCD and type A. One reason I waited was because I had heard of a couple people who were told they were having one gender and then delivered the other. It's harder to screw up the gender reveal when the genitals are out in the open!"

MICHELLE: "I wanted to find out with both pregnancies and could not fathom why someone would wait."

MELANIE: "We didn't find out. There are so few surprises left in life and we wanted baby's arrival to be a surprise. And we were! All the old wives' tales pointed to girl, but when baby arrived, we were blessed with a boy."

DANA: "We found out in advance both times. When my first was a girl, I wasn't surprised because I thought she was going to be a girl. When my second was a boy, I was genuinely surprised and cried (good cry) because I think it caught me off guard. I'm one of two girls myself and I think in my mind I was going to have two. Girls were all I knew! But he was a surprise to me! I always said if we had a third, we would not find out ahead of time, but we aren't having a third . . . which is a decision we made after having our boy! Ha!"

JILL: "We waited until they were born. And we got lucky and had one of each!"

SARAH: "I found out with both as soon as I could. I felt like there was so much else that was uncertain. I couldn't take one more surprise!"

TARA: "We found out at our 20-week ultrasound with both pregnancies. I was going to wait both times and didn't. With the first, I got really excited to decorate a nursery, so gave in and found out. I was set on waiting the second time and then I found out it was twins. That was enough of a surprise for us!"

LAURA: "We didn't want to know gender. If I'm being honest, I was afraid of having a boy and thought that if it was a boy, I'd be better off waiting until there was a baby in my arms to find out.

"During an ultrasound, the doctor said, 'I can't remember—do you know the gender?' And I said, 'No, we're waiting. Why do you ask?' And then she slipped and said, 'Because I can see "it" (meaning the penis). When I looked shocked, she said, 'Oops! Well, at least you'll know he's really well endowed!'

"I was a mess. I left, cried, freaked, regrouped, and planned a bris. Meanwhile, the other doctor in the ob-gyn group knew it was a girl! And she didn't tell us, she just let us think it was a boy for the next three months! Later, when I asked her why, she said, 'You didn't want to know the gender, so I didn't tell you.' But—but—but!

"Anyway, the rest is history. We had a girl, we were shocked and delighted, and we quickly converted the bris into a baby naming. We didn't have any girls' names chosen and had to talk that through fast, but otherwise it was just a fun and happy surprise."

Dear Bean Letters
Week 12, Gender

Dear Bean,

I've heard stories of people who wait until their baby is born to find out the gender. They say it's a thrill going into that delivery room not knowing whether they are coming out with a boy or a girl. What a great surprise!

I'm thinking these particular people don't fall as heavily into the "Control Freak" category of human beings as your Mommy. The thought of waiting another six months to find out your gender is more than my brain can take. And definitely more than my stomach can take.

You see, you are doing quite a number on that stomach. It's not a happy stomach. And it expresses its general contempt on a rather consistent basis. All day and all night I feel like I'm on the verge of puking. In fact, I spend most of that time taking very deep breaths and having very long conversations with myself about why it would not be a good idea to start puking. It's really a laugh a minute around here.

I know that these feelings and this nausea are happening because something awesome is taking place inside my body—I'm making you. And that makes me happy. Even when it also makes me want to put my head in a toilet.

So I try to concentrate on any and all things baby to keep myself from focusing too much on the head/toilet scenario. I visit the baby stores, I look online to research all the various items the Internet

➤

thinks I must own to be able to keep you alive. I study my pregnancy
tracker app every day to learn more about how you are developing.

These things make me happy.

But you know what would really make me happy? If I knew your
gender.

Because then I could distract myself with planning the nursery
or buying gender-specific clothes or coming up with a list of 50
possible names and 150 ways you might get made fun of for having
any of those names.

Basically, your gender will distract me for a little while and help
me stay focused on something besides vomiting. And anything that
takes my mind off of vomiting is a welcome addition to the day.

We are supposed to wait until our 20-week appointment to
find out your gender. That's the appointment where they measure
all your parts and check to make sure everything is progressing
well. The point of the appointment isn't specifically to find out your
gender, but it's the time when most parents get the news.

But I'm battling all-day morning sickness and I don't have the
patience to wait another eight weeks to find out whether you are a
boy or a girl. Mama knows a woman who does ultrasounds for high-
risk pregnancies and she agreed to let us come in after hours for
an ultrasound and to take a look at your bits. At twelve weeks your
bits are formed well enough that they are distinguishable; it's just a
matter of whether you are showing them off during the ultrasound.

I'm not going to lie; I hope you are a boy. I'm not sure why, I've
just always wanted a little boy. Maybe because I'm a tomboy myself
and I feel like I would be able to relate to a male child better. Maybe
because I'm frightened at the ball of emotions that will come my

way when a girl hits puberty. Maybe I just really, really like the adorable little man suits they make for boys. Who knows?

Mama wants a little boy too, but I think mostly because I've been so adamant in my desire for one. So we headed into the ultrasound hoping to see a penis.

When we started the ultrasound, you weren't giving up the goods, so we had to rummage around looking for them. Then we heard, "Oh, there we go. See that right there? Those lines? You are having a girl."

Mama looked at me with a sad look, as if I was going to be disappointed. And I started to cry. But not because I was disappointed. Not at all. I was so damn happy.

A little girl! My little girl!

I wasn't disappointed for even a split second. And I think I even forgot about puking for a little while.

I had a real live little girl growing in my belly. My daughter. My daughter. My daughter.

Awesome.

10

THE NAME YOU PICK COULD RUIN YOUR CHILD'S LIFE

Good luck with that

*W*HEN YOU ARE pregnant you are forced to make a lot of decisions regarding your upcoming child. All of these decisions seem really important. According to the Internet, the choices you make in regard to breastfeeding, diapers, and sleep training will have a profound effect on your kid's ability to become a functioning member of society. You don't want to mess anything up, because this is your child's future you are talking about!

But let's be honest here; most of the crap you are stressing about won't make or break your kid's future. The fact that you are stressing means that you are a caring parent who is going to look out for your offspring, and that matters more than whether your kid uses a pacifier.

But there is one thing that will without a doubt affect your baby for the rest of its life. And that thing is the name you pick for this little person. That name will follow your child into every classroom, every job interview, and every date for the rest of their life. Please do not send them into all those situations with a ridic- ulous name. Please.

Next up I'm going to break down some things you should consider when making the most important decision of your child's life. No pressure though.

PICK A NAME FOR AN ADULT, NOT A CHILD

A lot of times, people pick names that are adorable for a little girl who is all dressed up in a frilly skirt and has a bow the size of an eagle on her head. The name is delightful when typed in a calligraphy font on the birth announcement and all party invitations throughout childhood. But then the poor kid has to put that name on the top of a résumé and it looks like a Disney princess is applying for an upper-management position (not that a Disney princess couldn't kick the crap out of a management position; you see how they whip those talking animals into shape).

Or maybe you've given your boy a name that is perfect for yelling out when he's playing T-ball, but will get him laughed right out of a shareholder's meeting when he's 35.

I know you are thinking about your baby as, well, a baby, so it's hard to remember that eventually they are going to be an adult. In fact, they are going to be an adult for a hell of a lot longer than they are going to be wearing eagle-size bows or oversize batting helmets.

So you owe it to that adult to give them a name that they can take into all of life's situations without feeling self-conscious.

When I was picking my kids' names, I wanted to give them a name that would work no matter what they ended up doing with their lives. If Vivian wants to be a Supreme Court judge, she's all set. If she is the fun receptionist at an ad agency, she could go by Vivi. If she wants to be a bartender/artist, I feel like Viv will suit her well. Daniel could be Dan, Danny, or Daniel, depending on if he's a surfer, a teacher, or an insurance salesman.

The point is, you have no idea where these kids are going to go in life. It's your job to give them a name that will travel with them well, no matter where they end up.

THINK OF ALL THE WAYS THE CHILD WILL BE MADE FUN OF BECAUSE OF THIS NAME

While it's important to focus on giving your child an adult-ready name, you must also take into consideration the years they will spend lugging the moniker around other children. And other children are assholes.

Sit down with your list of names and spend a fair amount of time trying to come up with any and all ways other kids can turn that name into an insult. Dig deep. Access your inner asshole. Maybe call up a few actual assholes that you know, and ask them how they would make fun of each name.

This exercise won't allow you to magically discover the only name in the history of names that is taunt-proof, but it will help you eliminate some of the easier targets. Don't hand the bullies the gift of a name that rhymes with fart, for instance. Or any other bodily function, for that matter. Make the assholes work a little harder to make fun of your kid; maybe they'll get discouraged and move on to an easier name.

USE THE NAME WHEN TALKING
ABOUT THE BABY

Names can sound really great when you are picking them out of a book, or when you write them down next to your last name 100 times on a piece of paper. But when you actually start calling someone by the name, it can take on a different feel. I'm not sure why.

We went through quite a few names for Daniel before we landed on his final pick. Each time we changed his name, we would use that name when we were talking about him. "We have an appointment for Daniel's ultrasound next week." "Daniel is kicking like crazy today." "How do you think kids will make fun of the name 'Daniel'?" And so on.

Most of the names we tried out lost their luster after only a few days in the talking rotation. This was frustrating because each time we landed on a name, we were *sure* it was *the one*. Then 48 hours later, we were annoyed with the name and had to pick up the name book *again*.

This was a long process, but eventually we got to Daniel, tried it out, and didn't get annoyed throughout the weeks and months leading up to his birth. There's a small possibility we'd built up an annoyance tolerance while trying out the other 80 names he almost had, but either way, the name stuck.

A baby can feel very theoretical when it's still in your belly. Picking a name can also feel theoretical, as if you are in second grade and naming your kids during a game of MASH. I found that using the child's name in conversation helps bring them into reality before they are here, and also gives you a chance to course-correct a horrible name choice before it's too late.

TELL EVERYONE

Pregnant moms and dads are often given the advice to keep their child's name a secret until after the birth. The thought behind this advice is that sharing your name choice is going to open you up to criticism and leave you doubting yourself and your ability to name your own child. Everyone has an opinion and the last thing you need is every single one of those opinions, because there will be no way to somehow pick the one name that unanimously gets a thumbs-up from all the world. Without fail, there will be at least one person who says, "Oh, I knew someone with that name once. They ended up killing a family of four. But I'm sure it didn't have anything to do with the name!"

And then you are back to the baby book. Again.

While I understand the logic behind the advice to stay quiet, I have more faith in you than this advice gives you credit for. I think you are strong enough to wade through opinions and decide which ones are worth taking into consideration when making this choice.

We named Vivian after a grandmother and liked the name from the beginning, so we never really searched for an alternative. But with Daniel we had a more difficult time. It's really hard to find a solid name for a boy that will work when he's a man and isn't also the name of 250 million other boys.

As I mentioned before, we picked several names, tried them out, and tossed them to the side when they didn't work. Part of our "trying it out" process was sharing the name with other people.

The first name I loved was Elijah. I've always loved that name. It sounds like poetry to me. And it could be shrunk down to Eli or even E if necessary. But then I told my family and friends that I was going to name my son Elijah. And the looks on their faces told me that they weren't fans. I tried it out on other people, and I got similar looks. Eventually I moved on from Elijah to another 400 names in the course of four months.

I'm not someone who generally cares what other people think, so putting my child's name to vote seems a little out of character for me. But I am sending the kid out into the world with this name, and the reactions I'm getting to it are the same ones he's going to get. And that's something worth considering, for his sake.

I don't care if you once knew an Elijah who farted a lot or fired you from a job, that doesn't affect my kid. But if I get the same weird look from numerous people when they hear a name, I have to think he is also going to get that reaction throughout his life. And life is hard enough without having to brace yourself for judgment every time you say your damn name.

Keep in mind that this judgment can also come from a ridiculous spelling of a perfectly acceptable name. So, if you are planning on spelling your child's name in a way that seems super unique, but is really just super annoying, tell everyone about that plan as well. The looks you get when you explain the silent q or the "alternative spelling" will be the same looks your poor kid will get THEIR ENTIRE LIFE when they introduce themselves. Please take this into consideration and send your kid into the world with a name that is spelled correctly.

So take your name choice for a dry run a few months before delivery. See how it feels when you say it, see how other people respond when they hear it. Imagine it written on a name plate outside an office someday. Or as a punchline for an asshole kid's joke.

Do not take this lightly; the future of your child depends on it!

Again, no pressure.

Your Pregnancy Week by Week

HOW BIG IS YOUR BABY?

WEEK 16—CAN OF MOUNTAIN DEW

At 4½ inches from head to butt, your baby is the size of the Mountain Dew can I chose to stop drinking after I found out I was pregnant. When my doctor said I should add more greens to my diet, I somehow didn't think he was talking about fluorescent ones.

WEEK 17—TAKE-OUT CONTAINER

At about 5 inches tall, your baby is now as big as the many take-out containers in your fridge. Don't worry; "Kung Pao" means "Extra Healthy" in Chinese.

WEEK 18—SMALL MILK SHAKE WITH WHIPPED CREAM

At 5½ inches, your baby is about the size of a small milk shake from a drive-thru. You should probably go get one now. For research purposes.

WEEK 19—JACK IN THE BOX TACO

Your baby is about 6 inches from head to butt, which makes it about the size of a Jack in the Box taco. If you are like me, this conjures up a much clearer image than any of the fruit and vegetable references in your pregnancy app. It will also conjure up the idea of deep-frying a taco, which is a beautiful image indeed. 'Merica!

WEEK 20—BOX OF GIRL SCOUT COOKIES

At 6½ inches from head to rump, your baby is now about as big as a box of Girl Scout Thin Mint Cookies. This reminds me of when I was pregnant during Girl Scout Cookie season and I put out a Pregnant Lady Request for Thin Mints. Much like the Bat Signal, my Pregnant Lady Request was heeded by those near and far. I had three different people bring some to my house and one person send me some in the mail. It was delightful.

3RD QUARTER
(21–30 weeks)

Your Pregnancy Week by Week

HOW BIG IS YOUR BABY?

WEEK 21—REMOTE CONTROL

Your baby is 10½ inches from head to toe. No, your baby didn't actually grow 4 inches in one week—this week pregnancy apps and doctors start measuring baby from head to toe, instead of head to butt. Ten and a half inches is about how long one of those all-in-one remote controls can be. Currently, you use that remote control to access movies, TV, sports, documentaries, and comedy specials. After you have a baby, you will only use that remote to access kids' shows like *Caillou* and *Paw Patrol*. If you do not know what *Caillou* or *Paw Patrol* are, do not seek them out; they will find you soon enough. No need for you to be exposed any earlier than necessary.

WEEK 22—TOILET BOWL

Your baby is about 11 inches long, which is about as long as the opening to the toilet bowl you've been puking into since your first trimester.

WEEK 23—KITTEN

Your baby is a little over 11 inches long, which is about the size of a kitten that is a little over 11 inches long. I'm using a kitten as an example because they are soft and cuddly and adorable. And they are born pretty much potty trained, which makes them so much better than human babies.

WEEK 24—A RULER

I mean, if we are really trying to get a good idea of how long the child is, maybe you should just look at a damn ruler. Your baby is 12 inches long, which is how long a 12-inch ruler is, so that should give you a pretty accurate example.

WEEK 25—BROWNIES

Your baby is now 13½ inches, about the size of that pan of brownies you made last night for dessert and ended up eating for dinner instead.

Pregnancy WOD
MONTH 6

You are pretty deep into this training plan at this point. You may be sore, you may be weary, you should be frightened. But keep your head up. This is when we stop bathing. This is when it gets real.

1. Have an hour-long conversation with a potato (pick a cute one).

Babies are a lot of really great things. They are innocent, peaceful, and some may say they are proof of a higher being. But one thing they are not? Great conversationalists. Yes, they are able to get their point across, primarily via wailing and grimaces, but other than that they don't really hold up their end of a chat.

It is difficult to wrap your mind around exactly how much time you will spend silently staring at your baby once you bring them home. The staring will be a combination of love and the thousand-yard stare that comes when you've only slept four hours in three days. The silent part of the equation will be because there is only so much you can say to something that isn't saying anything back.

But talking to your baby is important, so practice having a conversation with the cutest potato you can find. Tell the potato how much you love them, about current events, and all the plans you have for their future (fried, twice-baked, hash browns, etc.). This will take up about three minutes, but you will still have the potato staring at you.

At this point you will need to dig deep and figure out ways to fill the potato silence. Make up songs, experiment with various fart sounds your mouth can produce, tell the potato the entire plot of

Breaking Bad, starting with episode one. Come up with these time burners now and your future spud will thank you for it.

2. Go two days without bathing.

This might not seem like a long time. And it isn't. We are just getting started.

3. Throw 375 various items on the floor of your living room.
Turn off the light. Grab your flour. Cross the living room without
dropping the flour or spraining your ankle.

If you take a look at your baby registry, you will probably notice that it has roughly 375 items on it. Inevitably each of those items will at some point make their way to your living room floor. They might not all go there at once, but over time they will slowly accumulate. You will be made horrifically aware of their accumulation when you are forced to navigate their obstacle course at 3 in the morning. While holding your fussy baby. You won't be able to turn on the light, because fussing is even louder with light shining on it. So you will hold on tight to the baby, taking step by risky step, hoping that the both of you aren't taken out by Aunt Joanne's thoughtful baby shower gift.

Practice this treacherous course while holding your flour baby, because unlike your real baby, your flour baby will actually break your fall when you trip and go flying to the ground the first few times.

IS THIS REALLY HAPPENING?

11

Don't worry if it doesn't feel real just yet

$\mathcal{P}$ REGNANCY IS THE most natural thing on the planet, they
say. I mean, what could be more natural than a living thing
growing inside your body? Sure, that is the setup for pretty much
every scary scene in every sci-fi movie you've ever watched, but
still, it's *natural*, don't worry. And when you are faced with this
totally natural occurrence, you are supposed to feel a surge of
maternal instincts, instead of the urge to run away flailing your
arms like they do in all those sci-fi movies.

But sometimes those maternal instincts don't seem to show
up in the way you anticipated they will. You are acting as an
incubator for a real live person. A person you will be tasked with
loving, protecting, and raising. You understand all of these things
on a logical level. But for some reason your emotions haven't
quite caught up. You don't *feel* like a mom. Even though you are
currently participating in a very significant mom activity.

Maybe you are going through the motions: making doctor's
appointments, picking out nursery furniture, stockpiling onesies
and bibs, pouring over every pregnancy and baby book you can
find. But as many motions as you go through, as happy as you

are, as big as that belly gets, all of this doesn't quite feel *real* yet. In some ways it may feel like a story you are telling yourself. A story about how you will have a baby someday. But it doesn't quite feel like today is that day.

But that's okay. Because today isn't actually the day you are having the baby. And until then—and maybe even after that—it's okay if all of this feels like a weird piece of performance art you are putting on. Just keep playing the part, and eventually you'll be holding a real live baby and you will never be short on *realness* ever again.

In my case I don't think I actually felt like a real mom until a couple of weeks after my first baby was born. It was around the time I finally started getting the hang of how to care for her. I knew I loved her, I knew she was mine, but only after the initial shock and awe of her arrival was I finally able to settle into the fact that I was actually a mom.

I was worried those first few weeks that I was missing some sort of mom gene. That I would forever just be playing the part and never quite feel like a real mom. But I gave myself some time and eventually something clicked in me, or her, or both of us.

So don't stress out if you are still having trouble wrapping your head around the sci-fi movie happening in your uterus. You aren't the only one who has ever felt this way. It's a weird, somewhat gross, and beautiful thing that is taking place. And I promise it all ends a lot better than those scary movies.

Moms on the Front Lines

MOM

I asked my MOFL when they actually felt like moms for the first time, and most of them were as emotionally vacant as I was until their baby made its appearance.

MICHELLE: "I felt like a mom the first night home. I was changing a diaper in the middle of the night while my husband was snoring. He didn't even hear the baby cry. That's when I knew it was all on me. Moms don't get a break; they are on call 24/7."

SARAH: "I didn't feel like a mom until Drew got here. During pregnancy it all just seemed so unnatural to have a person growing inside of you, even though it's the most normal thing in the world. I loved being pregnant, but it felt unnatural."

KAYSEE: "I felt like a mom once I could feel the baby moving around and I could see the 'bump'!"

MELANIE: "As he got older and continues to get older, I feel more and more like a mom. And I continue to be a learning mom who struggles with the littlest of things, but I love it."

TARA: "In my mind and heart, I earned the mom badge when they laid Drew on my chest for the first time in the delivery room."

MONICA: "The times I actually feel like a mom are when I bake chocolate chip cookies and have them ready for an after-school snack. When I actually prepare three real meals a day. When I am sitting at a soccer game or football game, cheering on my kids. I always know I am a mom but there are fun little moments when I feel like a 'mom.' Of course I felt like a mom when my babies were born and I was round-the-clock nourishing and nurturing them, but for some reason driving the minivan and preparing the four lunches every morning . . . those are the times I feel most like a mom."

Partner Corner
WHEN WAS IT REAL?

JASON: "When I walked out of the hospital with my first son in a car seat and the people in the hospital didn't come help us get him into the car. It was possibly the most terrifying moment of my life. That is when I realized I was always going to be a dad. This little life was going to look to me for everything and I'd better learn quick what to do."

KEVIN: "My twins were born three months early and had to stay in the NICU for two months. I didn't officially feel like a dad until we brought them home from the hospital, even though I spent hours upon hours with them before that."

MATT: "I felt like a dad the minute I knew she was pregnant. My responsibilities were taking care of Mom until the uterus exodus. When did it get real? When I had to pay the hospital bill. Actually, it always got real when the sex stopped for months, then ramped back up in month 8. . . . Maybe I should not have written that last part."

Dear Bean Letters
Week 25, Kick Counts

Dear Bean,

I've been told that I should be monitoring your kick counts. I should keep track of how long it takes for you to kick ten times in my belly. Apparently I am supposed to sit down, set a timer, and wait for you to kick ten times. If you don't kick ten times in two hours I need to contact my doctor.

I don't think I'm going to need to contact my doctor anytime soon.

You kick ten times before I'm even able to sit down and start the timer. I'm not sure what these other babies are doing during the two hours required to get their ten kicks in, but your primary uterine pastime is kicking everything in sight, as often as possible. You especially enjoy taking aim at my bladder, which is a special treat.

It took me a while to realize what your kicks felt like. Initially, when you were still pretty tiny, they felt like gas bubbles or a fluttering of sorts. Given the unfortunate situation in my stomach since being pregnant, I figured gas bubbles were just another pregnancy feature. But then the bubbles started getting bigger, less fluttery, more pop-y. Finally, because Mommy isn't so quick, I realized that they weren't bubbles at all, they were you, a tiny human being, assailing my insides.

Kick, kick, kick, tap, tap, tap.

I've loved feeling your kicks, all day, every day. I've loved them less all night, every night, but still they are a reminder that this pregnancy is real, that you are real, and that makes me happy.

I think one of the most exciting times so far was a night I was lying in bed reading a magazine. Mama was asleep next to me. You started to kick, because you must have gotten the message that I was in bed and thinking about going to sleep. But this time your kicks felt a little harder than before. I put my hand on my belly and sure enough, for the very first time, I could feel your kicks from the outside.

I immediately woke up Mama. She was frazzled and half asleep. I hit her repeatedly to bring her into focus.

"What? What's wrong?" she asked.

I grabbed her hand and put it on my belly. She was nervous, as if I was trying to tell her something bad. But then you came through and kick, kick, kick, tap, tap, tap. Her face lit up. "Is that . . . ?"

I smiled and nodded my head.

She sat up in bed and put both hands on my belly, finally being able to feel what I'd felt for weeks: "There's a baby in there!"

"I know!"

She gave my belly kisses and talked to you, the way she had so many times since we found out you were growing inside of me. But on this night you finally talked back a little.

Kick, kick, kick, tap, tap, tap.

Pregnancy WOD
MONTH 7

You can see the finish line just up around the bend. You've probably officially started to waddle and you may be peeing with alarming frequency while a human spends its days dancing on your bladder. I have taken your physical condition into consideration and devised these exercises accordingly. But what these lack in physical requirements they more than make up in psychological tests. You didn't think you'd get off that easy, did you?

1. Go three days without bathing.

Or changing your clothes.

2. Make a hasty exit from a restaurant.

If you are anything like me, you enjoy a meal cooked by someone else. Especially when that someone else works in a nice restaurant. Like me, you may spend more than an average amount of time eating in restaurants because cooking is hard. Or at least you think it is, because to be honest, you've never really tried it.

Of course you understand that kids will slow down the frequency of your restaurant visits, but you are confident that you will have children who behave well in restaurants and will be comfortable with visiting them often.

Aren't you adorable.

To prepare for your post-baby restaurant experiences, you are going to have to make some minor adjustments to the way you

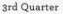

dine out. The first adjustment is the time you are allowed to stay in the restaurant. No, there isn't a set amount of time that children behave in a restaurant setting, and that is what makes this game so much fun. You may have an hour, you may have three and a half minutes—no one knows for sure. Even your baby doesn't know. They can be doing fine in the restaurant and then all of a sudden a waiter looks at them the wrong way and it will signal to their brain that it is time to get the hell out of this establishment. The signal will in turn reach your brain via a high-pitched wail.

When that wail comes, no matter when it comes, your time is up. Please exit immediately, do not wait for to-go boxes, do not exchange pleasantries with the waiter. Throw cash in the general direction of someone who looks like they work at the restaurant, and flee the scene.

The best way to prepare for this new restaurant experience is to shake off your old dining routine before the baby joins you. No more dilly-dallying over appetizers and beverages. Study the menu in advance and order as soon as you are seated. When your food arrives, ask for a to-go box, because you may be required to turn this dine-in to a take-out order at a moment's notice. Also, immediately ask for your check. Pay it before you have even completed your meal. That way, you are free to flee whenever the wailing begins. Don't even bother looking at that dessert tray. You are years away from seeing another restaurant dessert; say good-bye to them now and forget all the good times you've shared. It's easier that way.

Before you leave the restaurant, throw 75 napkins on the table and half of your food on the floor, so you can get a good idea of

THE SH!T NO ONE TELLS YOU

the mess you will be leaving behind from now on. Because of this, you will also need to go back and increase your tip amount by an additional 15 percent.

And on the way home, maybe buy a cookbook . . .

3. When you get up in the morning, look at yourself in the mirror, throw on a little makeup (optional), run a brush through your hair (also optional), and decide that you are now ready to go about your day. Do not change out of your pajamas, even if you are leaving the house.

For the first months of new motherhood, you will give not one single shit what you look like while inside of your house. Eventually that lack of shits will grow to include your appearance outside of the house as well. You will be too tired and overwhelmed to spend the time and five gallons of concealer it would take to try to bring your face back to life, so you will regularly head out into the world looking alarmingly similar to how you looked when you got out of bed that morning (and to someone in need of professional psychological help).

This WOD is as much for your benefit as it is for those around you. All of you need to get used to your upcoming change of appearance and being eased into it will help everyone practice their individual reactions to it. Seeing looks of horror slide across people's faces when you enter the room can be really hard on your postpartum brain, so get those looks out of the way now when you still have the emotional strength to deal with it.

4. Close your eyes. Have a friend or family member grab the most disgusting thing they can find. Open your eyes as they throw this disgusting thing at you. Put your hands out and catch the thing, no questions asked.

Before becoming a parent it is human nature to avoid gross things. This is because gross things are, well, gross. And who wants to be around them? No one. And there's also not anyone who wants to touch the gross things. Because we aren't animals.

Once you enter parenthood, quite a few areas of your brain cease to operate at full capacity. The most significant alteration happens to the part of your brain in charge of disgust. Initially you will be quite alarmed by the various liquids coming out of your baby, and you will be absolutely horrified by how much of that liquid you are coming into direct contact with. But over time you will build up a tolerance for the disgusting things coming out of your child. Eventually parenting will wear you down to the point where putting your hands out to catch vomit and/or feces will seem like a completely logical reflex.

This WOD will help you work on those reflexes before your child arrives, so you can avoid running off in horror at the sight of your baby's first shit explosion. Start this WOD by having your assistant throw mildly offensive things at you (think cottage cheese or sour milk), and gradually work your way up to dog poop.

Also, as you get better at this WOD have your assistant throw disgusting things at you without prior notice. As a parent you need to always be on high alert and ready to catch bodily fluids. This is one of the more magical parts of parenting; you might as well get used to it now.

12

THE REGISTRY YOU REALLY NEED

Make this list, check it twice

I WAS GOING TO tell you about all the stuff that you are inevitably going to put on your baby registry, and how little of that stuff you will ever actually need. Or how little of it you or your child will use for more than four minutes.

I was also going to go on and on about the ridiculous amounts of cash we all spend on baby whatnots, in some misguided belief that the more whatnots we have, the easier our baby-raising will be. I was going to tell you that all you really need is a bunch of diapers, onesies, and some Tupperware® (because for some reason babies are endlessly entertained by Tupperware).

But then I realized it's pretty much impossible to convince an expectant mother to go easy on her baby registry. Even if she has good intentions she'll most likely be powerless to control herself once she's let loose inside of Babies "R" Us with that little registry gun they give you. You start off simply with a pack of diapers here and some bibs there. Then before you know it, you are drunk on power and streaking through the aisles with your gun out, blindly zapping every item you pass. It happens.

I don't want to begrudge anyone of her duly earned excitement, so I say register with abandon. If friends and family are going to bring you gifts, great! They can choose from the 14 pages of registry items you helpfully suggested.

But after that, when the gifts have dwindled, and it's time to make your own purchasing choices, I would recommend lowering your requirements on acceptable baby whatnots. Secondhand baby stuff is often damn near firsthand, because babies only use their whatnots for three minutes before growing out of them or growing bored with them. Buy and accept and seek out all secondhand baby stuff that you can find. Your bank account will thank you for it.

While I know there is no way to talk you out of a ridiculously bloated baby registry, I do feel like it's my responsibility to talk to you into another kind of registry. One that is equally, if not more, important. Because it will include all the things you really need. I like to call this list *The Mommy Registry*.

With all of your Babies "R" Us registry gun shenanigans, it's likely that you've completely overlooked the things you will actually need to survive motherhood. And since Babies "R" Us doesn't offer bulk discounts on wine, I'm pretty sure you have to head to another store to complete *The Mommy Registry*.

THE MOMMY REGISTRY
*(some, but not all, of the items needed
for Mommy survival)*

Larger Purse

The amount of accessories and doodads needed to keep your child alive and entertained is hard to adequately explain. When your baby is brand-new, a lot of his or her necessities will be carried around in your overpriced diaper bag. But even then, you'll find that your purse becomes the final resting place for countless baby-related items.

As your child gets older you will stop using the diaper bag and your poor purse will be solely responsible for transporting all of your parenting requirements. As I type this, my purse is full of granola bars, underwear, suckers, stickers, fruit snacks, tissues (used and new), hand sanitizer, party invitations (from months ago), and an empty juice box. I think I might have a wallet in there somewhere as well.

My kids are no longer babies, so my current purse is actually quite a bit lighter than it was in the past.

So when you are buying your fancy new diaper bag, go ahead and grab a purse the size of your torso as well. That purse will be responsible for transporting everything required to parent your child when you are outside of your house. You better make sure it has a really strong strap.

Bladder Leakage Panty Pads

Light bladder leakage (LBL) is a thing. It has an acronym. It happens to women who have given birth. And these pads will help curb some possible embarrassment. Glamour is your new middle name.

Push-up Bra

Take a glimpse at those wonderful boobs of yours. Look at them sitting up so high and mighty. They have no idea what is coming their way. Or how far they will tumble from their current berth. Help them out and grab a nice push-up bra now, before they start their inevitable trek down toward your navel. Once they are there, you will be happy that you have a handy transportation device to bring them back up to their previous glory.

Tankini

A tankini is a like a bikini, except the top part is long and does everything it can to keep your middle section under wraps. It's really doing the Lord's work.

Once you have a baby, your stomach muscles usually go on strike. You went and stretched everything out, and they aren't in the mood to put it all back together the way it looked before. Your tankini understands this struggle and is here to help you deal with it.

All the Caffeine

As soon as you become a parent, you will be thrust into a sleep-deprived haze that will last for approximately two decades. You will slowly build up a tolerance for this haze and eventually be able to perform most of your day to day activities despite the limited capabilities of your tired brain. And by "build up a tolerance" I mean "develop a caffeine addiction."

Some people like their caffeine in coffee form; some people like it in Red Bull form; some people, like me, consume Mountain Dew in quantities that are probably not recommended by anyone who has ever read the ingredients or seen the color of Mountain Dew. We all do what we can to get by.

Go to 7-Eleven, grab one of those drink cups that is big enough to hold a small child (coincidence?), buy it, and keep it on hand to transport any and all caffeine your body will require once you become a parent.

Dry Shampoo

It should be no secret that regular bathing habits are soon to be a distant memory for you.

Dry shampoo lets you "shampoo" your hair without having to do all that silly disrobing, standing under warm, refreshing water, and lathering up the rest of your body with soap. Because who has time for such things? (You should probably stock up on deodorant too . . .)

Hair Ties

As you might have gathered from the last item, you aren't always going to get around to doing your hair every day.

Stock up on hair ties and stash them in various parts of your home. Please be warned that hair ties, taking a cue from socks, regularly run away from you and your home, never to be heard from again. They leave without warning, and often when you need them most.

Don't be left stranded by their abandonment—buy them in bulk before it's too late.

Yoga Pants

I'm not even sure what yoga pants are, since I've only done yoga one time and am pretty sure I was wearing the wrong pants (because I'm sure the right pants would have made me much better at yoga). But it seems as though every mom rambles on about her beloved yoga pants, so you should probably grab some.

My version of yoga pants are a comfortable pair of loose black pants that could reasonably be considered something someone might wear if she was so inclined as to twist her body into yoga poses. They are comfy and stain resistant, and I've been wearing them every day for going on six years.

Find some comfy pants of your own and buy a few pairs. If you really want to excel at the Mommy game, you should consider getting yoga pants with at least a tiny pattern on them. This pattern will help disguise the many stains your pants will harbor before you finally throw them in the wash. The better the pattern, the less laundry you have to do. Choose wisely.

Multi-Pack of Car Washes

The carwash by my house offers a deep discount if you purchase a multi-pack of car washes in advance. I recommend you find a similar deal and get multi-packs of the multi-packs. The impending mess inside your car is not something you will be able to handle by yourself; you are not a miracle worker. You will regularly need someone with access to an industrial-strength vacuum to help you. They are also going to need roughly 14 gallons of professional cleaning solution. Tip these people well, if they make it out alive.

- -

Stain Stick and Stain Spray in Bulk

I feel like this is self-explanatory. Or at least it will be very soon.

Six-Pack of Wine Holder

If you are breastfeeding, then you are obviously going to need to hold off on consuming the wine in this six-pack, but that doesn't mean you can't get it all ready for the day after your little bundle of joy finally releases control of your nipples, and your liver.

Under-Eye Cream

And possibly the number of a very good plastic surgeon.

Post-it Notes

Before you have kids your brain may be a place of wonder and order. You may keep several running lists at one time, you may have an extensive and well-versed vocabulary, you may never walk into a room and have no idea what the hell you are doing there.

Unfortunately, your lease on that brain is just about up. And it will be replaced by a much more tired model. That model isn't going to be great with lists or vocabulary or dates. Plan ahead for this system malfunction by buying the biggest package of Post-it notes that you can find.

Once you have your baby, keep these Post-it notes within arm's reach at all times. When a thought enters your head you should immediately jot it down on a Post-it note, because immediately after that the thought will take leave of your brain, never to return.

Napkins

I don't think I was really prepared for the amount of napkins I would blow through once I had kids. Grab all the napkins you can find and fill your pantry with them. And then fill another room. And that will still not be enough napkins. There are never enough napkins.

Door Locks

I asked my MOFL what items they would recommend for *The Mommy Registry* and Amy recommended door locks. I asked her if she meant door locks for the kid's door or for her door. She responded, "All the doors. So you can isolate yourself at any time." Listen to Amy.

Partner Corner

JEREMY: "All the nursery stuff and baby crap drove me nuts more than anything. Since I don't have baby juices raging through my veins, I can logically look at the latest 'must-have' rubber baby junk and go, 'Nah, we don't need that.' But there is no arguing with a hormone-raging prego-chick. You just resign yourself that you are going to buy all this crap, and never use it, then throw or give it away."

"And it Costs. So. Damn. Much. Money.

"I swear to God, if you want to be a millionaire, design some baby doodad, paint it blue and pink, rub newborn smell on it, market it in all the 'mom forums,' and wait for the profit to roll in. By the time the ex-expecting mothers realize it wasn't necessary, they are diligently trying to pawn it off on the next generation of up-and-coming moms to recoup some of the mortgage-busting money that was spent on it in hopes of appeasing their still annoyed husbands."

Partner Corner
MOMMY AND MAMA

KRISTA (who gave birth to her first two sons, and her partner gave birth to her third): "I feel so grateful to have had both experiences. They are so different. With my first two, it was happening to me. As a partner to a woman going through it, especially as a lesbian mom who had experienced it herself, it was challenging. We were not seen as lesbians by those around us. If you're a pregnant woman, you're obviously straight. I could have had my hand in her pants, and right to her face, someone, a sales clerk, a nosy parent, a stranger, would say, 'Your husband must be so excited,' or 'Is this for your husband?' Even in the maternity store, I was her 'good friend.' It infuriated me and made me feel invisible as a new and expectant mom."

BECKY: "Being in a same sex/lesbian/gay relationship and trying for kids is both cool and really hard. As women the cool part was deciding who would have the kids. Had I not been diabetic, I probably would have jumped at the opportunity. But I am diabetic, so we choose Dawn instead. And getting pregnant was very scientific for us. There was nothing romantic about it.

"Because I didn't carry the babies, it meant my DNA was not involved. There was never even a little chance that these babies would look like me. That was hard. But I'm so glad we choose Dawn to carry them. They are adorable and stubborn and funny and I don't feel like I love them any less for not having carried them. I feel like they are my babies, because they are.

"Overall I would say being the girl in the dad role is a hard gig. You have to have a pretty thick skin to be able to handle not having given birth like every other mom you are friends with. You have to have confidence to be able to talk with other moms because you didn't have that experience. You're like a dude, but not really. I've been lucky and feel like my girlfriends always let me into the mom conversation even though I didn't fully earn that right. But I love our kids so much and that's probably all you really need to be in the Mom Club."

13

IT'S TIME TO HUDDLE UP

Setting a post-baby game plan

*A*LOT OF PLANNING happens during pregnancy. There is a new baby on the way and parents have to prepare in numerous ways. Where are they going to put the baby? What are they going to feed the baby? What are they going to name the baby? How in the hell are they going to survive a baby when they were worn out by dog-sitting their cousin's labradoodle for three days last summer?

There's a lot to think about. And I hate to add to the list, but a few very important things often don't get much attention during pregnancy and then turn out to be very important once the baby is here. And once the baby is here is a terrible time to be hashing out important issues.

I know you've thought at great length about the color of the nursery and whether to go with cloth or disposable diapers, but it's time to huddle up and figure out some other key details as well. This is a two-person huddle, so grab your partner and settle in for some planning.

One of the biggest mistakes couples can make when heading into parenting is to blindly assume that the two of them are on the same page about everything regarding their new baby. Yes, you two love each other. Yes, you seem to have similar beliefs and morals and tastes. But that in no way guarantees that you have the same expectations for how things are going to go down once a baby barrels into your home.

So get together now and have a chat about what you are expecting of each other post-baby-barrel. This chat may go very smoothly because of course you are of one mind about how you'll raise your impending spawn. Or this chat may reveal some appalling differences in expectations, because it turns out you two are actually different people with different points of view. It could go either way, really.

In the case of the appalling differences, it is much better to have those differences exposed and discussed now, instead of discovering them at 3 AM while holding a two-day-old screaming baby. Trust me.

Partner Corner
PART 1

I usually put the Partner Corners at the end of the chapter, but the following message needs to be up front and clear. Yes, it's important for couples to huddle up and work out the details of their lives post-baby, but there are some things a partner needs to know independent of any family meeting.

⟩

Dear partners,

Your Baby Mama is going to be a mess, and your baby is going to be a completely foreign object to both of you. You can't help her hormones, and you might not even be very effective in helping with the actual baby. But you can do little things to help keep the wheels on during this trying time (or at least a couple of the wheels on, because, let's be honest, you aren't a miracle worker).

If she is stuck breastfeeding for 23 hours out of her day, then you need to step up and take care of the things she can't do with a human attached to her boob. Do the many loads of laundry that need to be done every day, tackle that pile of dishes in the sink, make some meals for the two of you. Also, keep her breastfeeding station well stocked with water, magazines, blankets, pillows, snacks, iPads, and remotes so that she doesn't go completely insane while chained to a chair for hours.

If she's comfortable with it, encourage your Baby Mama to pump between feedings, so that you can try bottle-feeding the baby to alleviate a little of the pressure on her.

In general, your main goal is to never let her feel as if she is the only one suffering. They say misery loves company, but in this case misery will just get really pissed off if her company is showing any signs of comfort. If you are relaxing on the couch, you'd best be holding a sleeping baby. If Mommy doesn't bathe, no one bathes. And probably don't even consider asking whether it's okay for you to head out with your buddies "because it's kinda boring here." That's a very good way to make sure things get very un-boring very quickly. And by "un-boring" I mean filled with an "onslaught of hormonal rage."

Consider yourself warned, dear partners.

Now, let's get into some of the issues you should probably hash out before your baby arrives. For everyone's sake.

Baby Duties

A lot of couples run into disagreements early on because they never actually discussed the expectations each of them had for how they were going to tackle different baby duties. This seems like pretty basic stuff, but it can become a pretty heated conversation when these differences present themselves.

Even if Mom is taking care of feeding the child, there are still many more tasks that can be split up. How will you deal with middle-of-the-night (or middle-of-the-afternoon, for that matter) screaming fits that aren't cured by feeding? Diaper changes? Bathing? Or just hanging out with the baby during non-feeding, non-crying, non-sleeping time (this is not *a lot* of time at the beginning, but it's still worth talking about).

I've known several new moms who didn't realize they were in a 1950s marriage until after they came home with their new baby. These women had husbands who assumed that pretty much all of the baby duties fell on the shoulders of their wives. I'll let you guess how well that assumption worked out for those husbands.

In our house Becky was in charge of bathing both of the kids when they were brand-new. It was a short time each day that she got some real one on one time with them. I would collapse on the couch and enjoy some solitude while Becky splashed water on the baby and asked, "Soooo, how was your day?" Every day. She sang songs, "brushed" their teeth, and cleaned their little bodies. It was nice for her to feel connected to the babies and for me to have a moment when they weren't connected to my boob.

- -

During your pre-baby huddle, you need to have an open conversation about how each of you are expecting this task-management adventure to go. Do this with the understanding that neither of you really has any idea what shit is coming your way. But that doesn't mean you can't get some basic rules down on paper. Commit to sharing parenting responsibilities. Commit to communicating about what those responsibilities are as the child grows and needs different things. Commit to being vocal about what each of you needs independent of the baby. Commit to being gentle with each other as you both deal with the exhaustion and disorientation that comes with new parenthood.

While you're negotiating, I recommend discounting "lack of experience" as a reason for opting out of any task. Every parent has to fill the parenting position to the best of their abilities, and it's obviously understood that this will involve a lot of on the job training.

Sleep

Technically sleep (or lack thereof) falls under the Baby Duties heading, but I'm calling it out because you'll find it at the root of many early parenting squabbles. Even if sleep isn't the exact cause of your fight, odds are fatigue is playing a significant role.

There is no way to adequately prepare yourself for the lack of sleep your life will include once that life also includes a baby. So your huddle is useless in that regard. But you can discuss your upcoming change in sleep patterns and agree to be conscious of sharing the load.

Recently a new (tired) mom told me about feeding her son in the middle of the night. She was nursing in a rocking chair in her room. From this rocking chair, she could see her husband sleeping soundly in bed. This enraged her. She yelled at her husband to wake up. He was startled awake and was very confused. He wondered why he needed to be awake while she was breastfeeding. What was the point? She screamed, "If I'm awake, you have to be awake!" And so then everyone was awake.

Honestly, there's not much partners can do to alleviate the lack of sleep breastfeeding mothers get. But they can at least try to minimize the suffering. In my house Becky would get up each time one of the babies needed to feed in the middle of the night. She would get the baby out of its crib, change its diaper, get it re-dressed, and present it to me for feeding. All I would have to do is stumble down the hallway and collapse in the nursery chair. After she handed me the baby, she'd double-check that I had a large cup of water and anything else I needed before she headed back to bed.

No, she wasn't up for as long as I was, and her body wasn't single-handedly keeping a baby alive, but I appreciated that she climbed out of bed several times a night to help me get the baby changed and fed. It gave me five extra minutes to stay horizontal, and I felt a stronger solidarity with her in the morning. Trust me, if you are the partner to a nursing mom, the last thing you want is to look well rested in the morning. That is not going to end well for you.

Another thing to keep in mind is that not all baby crying can be solved by shoving a boob in its face. There were plenty of times when my babies decided that crying for hours on end was a delightful way to pass the middle of the night hours. My magical boobs wouldn't help this crying and I needed reinforcements.

During these times Becky and I would trade off bouncing the irate baby around the house, trying to calm it down. She would bounce for an hour or two while I slept, and then we'd switch. This not only alleviated some of the pressure on me, but also gave Becky a chance to bond with the babies.

A lot of times men will shy away from comforting their babies, because they feel like their wife is so much better at it. That means that the wife takes over comforting the baby when it's fussy, and then eventually she becomes the only one who can comfort the fussy baby. See how that works out?

In my relationship I was definitely less comfortable with babies than Becky was. She had been around babies her whole life and instinctively knew what to do with them. I, on the other hand, was terrified of infants and had made it a point to avoid them at all costs. When my first newborn arrived, I expected a maternal switch to click on and send waves of mommy instincts through my veins. That did not happen.

In the beginning when my baby cried or fussed, I immediately handed her over to Becky, because she knew what to do. Unfortunately, I was the keeper of the magic boobs, so there were a lot of times when I wasn't able to simply hand the baby off and run screaming into the night.

When I think back on that time, I realize how grateful I am that I breastfed Vivian. It forced me to get to know her. It left me alone with her for hours on end, hours I spent figuring out how to operate a newborn.

This is all to say that neither partner is going to get good at parenting by handing the child off when the parenting gets difficult. If you are the one who is more comfortable with babies, make it a point to force your partner to learn. Hand them the baby and disappear for a while (under a comforter in bed, perhaps?). Don't judge their clumsy beginnings; let them make mistakes and stumble through figuring out how to operate your child.

If you are the less experienced partner, force yourself to take the screaming baby, even when every part of you is uncomfortable with the idea. You will not break the baby. And it's already screaming, so how much worse can it get?

Agreeing early on that you will share the baby load, especially in those endless nighttime hours, will cut down on resentment and will ensure that you both are equally exhausted, as it should be.

House Duties

While it will feel like your new baby has taken over your entire life, there will also be other matters that still need tending to. For instance, this child will produce an incomprehensible amount of laundry. And their arrival in your house will somehow trigger a huge, permanent pile of dishes in your sink. I'm not sure of the science behind either of these facts, but I know them to be true.

Even though, again, it turns out we aren't living in the 1950s, a lot of couples have issues when it comes to dividing up the various house duties of the house they are both residing in.

Kaysee, one of my MOFL, said her husband was extremely helpful and involved in the care of all of her babies but, "Looking back, I wish I would have laid more groundwork for the other household chores. Sometimes the cooking, grocery shopping, and laundry can become overwhelming. Especially if you are working at all. I think the 'roles' need to be defined early on."

This is another subject that may seem silly to discuss in advance, because of course each partner is going to help out with keeping their home in running order. I mean really. But just for shits and giggles, maybe add a list of household chores to your pre-baby negotiations and agree to split them up post-baby. In the early days, if one partner is spending most of her time as a feeding machine for the child, then it would seem more than a little bit fair if her partner picked up most of the household duties. As the baby gets older, keep this conversation going and make sure that you both continue to share the load when it comes to keeping your house running.

Dealing with different maternity and/or paternity leaves can complicate the distribution of duties, but that should be discussed before the baby arrives as well. It's easy to assume that one partner going back to work automatically means that the other partner is solely responsible for the baby and the house. I would highly recommend avoiding this assumption if you happen to be the partner returning to work first.

Yes, everyone is aware that you have to get up and go to work tomorrow. But we are also aware that you agreed to bring a new person into the world and in doing so agreed to help care for that person. So get your ass out of bed and help with your child. You can nap on your lunch break tomorrow.

The distribution of house duties can get especially tricky if one parent is working less or staying home full-time with the child. There have been many men who have walked into their house after work, looked around at the mess, and asked, "What have you been *doing* all day?" These men have barely survived to tell the tale.

If you are the partner who is working more, it is in your best interest to come home with the assumption that your second shift of the day is starting. How can you help? Can you make dinner? Can you clean up the kitchen? Can you take the baby so that your partner can lock themselves in the bathroom for a half hour and decompress from a day spent with an infant? If I were you, I would assume the answer is always: All of the above.

Another suggestion I have in this area is to look into the costs of hiring a housekeeper. I'm not kidding. Having a housekeeper come reset your home once or twice a month is like having those magical animals from Disney movies come shine the inside of your house. It'll make your soul so happy you may even whistle a little tune.

You may think you don't have the money for a housekeeper in your budget, but you'd be surprised how cheap they can be, especially if they are only coming once or twice a month. Put the expense in the health-care category of your budget. Because it will aid in the health of your brain tremendously.

Family and Friends

Bringing a new baby home is one of the most stressful times in a person's life. And for some reason it's also the time when everyone wants to come over and visit. These people mean well, but sometimes they are a giant pain in the ass.

I've heard horror stories of mothers-in-law who insist on moving in to "help" with the baby, and then never leave. Or friends who "pop in" unannounced and stay through dinner (that they don't help make).

There's no way to know for sure how you are going to feel about visitors (or imposing in-laws) until you are knee-deep in diapers and hormones, but it's still a good idea to set some boundaries beforehand.

Get out your paper and pencil, because this should be documented. Which family and friends do you want to come visit you at the hospital? Make a list. That's right, write it down. Then hand it to your partner.

It will be the partner's job to enforce that list. "Oh, you know, they are both sleeping right now; it's not a great time for a visit. How about we connect once we get home, or maybe in four years?" Also, be prepared to alter that list down to zero if you aren't feeling up for visitors. Yes, this may hurt some feelings, but they'll get over it.

Once you head home, your dance card will be full of people wanting to give the baby a twirl. Some days, you may feel like opening up the welcome gates; and others you may want to hide in the closet and ignore any and all knocks at the door. It might be a good idea to warn any particularly sensitive well-wishers (cough, mother-in-law, cough) that you may need some space for a little while. Assure them now that you love them and value them, but you cannot be held accountable for becoming a hormonal hermit after you have your baby. If you're uncomfortable, get your partner to do it. You're the one who carried the baby for nine months—your partner can endure the nine seconds it takes to keep an overeager well-wisher away.

Conversely, there will be friends and family who go out of their way to keep their distance, even though they want nothing more than to snuggle your child for hours. These people may not want to impose and you may get your feelings hurt because they aren't clamoring to come over. Let the important people in your life know in advance that you want them to come see the baby, then follow up once you are feeling social.

(Another) Partner Corner

I reached out to my MOFL to ask them how their partners had contributed when their babies were brand-new. Many said their husbands stepped up in a big way to help out, whereas others bemoaned their partner's lack of involvement.

But the response I got from Sarah was the one I thought you partners should hear. I remembered visiting Sarah when her first baby was only a couple of weeks old. She was exhausted and overwhelmed. During the visit I noticed her husband change the baby's diaper several times. When I complimented him on it, he said he was changing all the diapers; it was the least he could do, because she grew a baby and pushed it out. I remember thinking this was very cute.

I reminded Sarah about these diaper changes and she said, "Yes, he did! With my first baby, I don't think I changed a diaper at all until he was, like, three weeks old. He also took one feeding a night so I could at least get a four-hour stretch of sleep. He did lots of sweet things. However, at the time it didn't feel that way! Damn hormones!"

I'm sharing Sarah's thoughts with you, dear partners, because it's important for you to know that even if you do everything right, make concerted efforts to contribute, and go out of your way to help, the odds are your Baby Mama might not heap praise on you, or even express gratitude. So don't expect a gold star for your efforts.

But don't let this deter you from doing the right thing. Parenting in general is a pretty thankless task, so you should get used to it right out of the gate.

Your Pregnancy Week by Week

HOW BIG IS YOUR BABY?

WEEK 26—COTTON CANDY
At about 14 inches, your baby is about the size of a soft and fluffy stick of cotton candy. Doesn't it make you feel better about childbirth to think about your baby as soft and fluffy?

WEEK 27—CAULIFLOWER?
My pregnancy apps say that your baby is the size of cauliflower at 27 weeks. But they also say that your baby is 14½ inches long. I don't actually eat cauliflower and am morally opposed to the rash of people trying to incorporate it into everyday life (stop it with the cauliflower pizza, please), but I don't recall cauliflower being 14½ inches big. Maybe your baby is huddled up into a cauliflower ball?

WEEK 28—REALLY CUTE BOOTS
You know those really cute boots women wear? The ones that zip all the way up the side and end just below her knee? She rocks them with a cute skirt, à la Kalinda on *The Good Wife*? Your baby, at about 15 inches long from head to toe, is about as long as those boots. If you have any of those boots, you should wear them now. Jam your swollen feet into them and take them for a spin. Because they will be replaced by very sensible shoes/maybe even just slippers after you bring home a newborn.

WEEK 29—BALLOON
Your baby is a little over 15 inches long this week, which is about the size of your average balloon. Except your balloon, and your belly, aren't done inflating just yet.

WEEK 30—TINY ANIMALS
At about 15¾ inches from head to toe, your baby is now much closer in size to living animals found in the wild than to fruit or vegetables found in the produce section.

4TH QUARTER
(31–40 weeks)

Your Pregnancy Week by Week

HOW BIG IS YOUR BABY?

WEEKS 31–34—THIS IS GETTING OUT OF HAND

This is the time in your pregnancy when knowing the size of the baby stops being helpful and starts getting alarming. Sure, it's great that your fetus is growing and developing on schedule. But there aren't that many days left on the calendar before you will have to negotiate that growing child out of you. And it's ever-increasing size is ever increasingly stressing you out.

Your baby is ranging from 16 to 18 inches these weeks and I'm not a fan of any of the produce comparisons these sizes bring along. Maybe think about a soft loaf of bread. Or four rolls of toilet paper stacked on top of one another.

Or don't. Instead, why don't you go eat something with lots of calories or reorganize the nursery for the 734th time? These are much more positive uses of your time.

Pregnancy WOD
MONTH 8

All right, people. It's almost go time. You're huge, you're uncomfortable, and this baby thing is becoming more real by the second. But don't worry! You're prepared! You've mastered your Pregnancy WOD and you are in the homestretch now. Do this last set of workouts and you will officially earn your "Ready for All the Shit Coming My Way" certificate. It will be the envy of all parents who hear of your feat.

1. Spill milk on your shirt in the morning. Walk around the rest of the day (and maybe the next day) wearing the stained shirt.

As you can tell by our previous months' WODs, bathing and personal appearance will plummet down your list of things to care about once you have a baby. On the flip side, think of all the time you will save when you stop changing your clothes every day. What a life hack!

Stains on clothes are usually a reason to implement one of those laborious outfit changes, but soon you will pay no attention to stifling social norms such as this.

All babies do is stain clothes. Their own and those of everyone in their general vicinity. They poop, pee, spit up, and throw food. If you were to change your clothes every time they were stained by a baby, you would burn through your wardrobe by day three. And then you'll be left to breastfeed while wearing that old bridesmaid's dress that has been buried in the back of your closet for six years. And no one needs to see that.

>

When you first tackle this WOD, start with only a milk stain. Then slowly add more stains (food and bodily fluids) to your shirt and build up your tolerance for wearing soiled clothing. Finally break down and change your outfit when people physically remove themselves from your presence because of your smell.

2. Go to Chuck E. Cheese on a Saturday afternoon, during prime birthday party time. Put on a party hat and join one of the celebrations. That's right, get up in the thick of the singing, screaming, germ spreading, and crappy pizza. Stay as long as you can handle it. Then stay another hour.

We are getting down to the wire here, your tolerance for noise and chaos needs to be on point. If there aren't at least three different parties occurring when you visit Chuck E. Cheese come back at a later time. This is no time for slacking.

3. Set off the alarm in your house. Then make an important phone call.

Any and all phone calls after you have children will become an exercise in tolerance for both yourself and anyone who has the misfortune of having to speak to you. Trying to having a conversation while a blaring alarm goes off in the background is about as close as you are going to get to practicing for phone calls with a baby anywhere near you.

The good news is that it'll be a while until the baby can chase after you, so also practice fleeing into a closet and building a soundproof fortress out of sweatshirts, parkas, and shoe boxes.

THE SH!T NO ONE TELLS YOU

While you're there, set up a comfortable area for yourself, this will be where you conduct most of your phone calls as a parent.

While I don't want to deter you from mastering this WOD, I will also note that most parents give up on phone calls as a means of communication on about day three of parenting. In addition to the above alarm/closet scenario, you should also practice ignoring any and all calls that come in. Train your people now to expect only text messages from you for the next three to five years.

4. If you plan to breastfeed: Ask a friend to grab your boobs and pull them halfway across the room.

Do this several times a day so you aren't completely horrified by what a breast pump does to your body.

4a. If you plan to bottle-feed: Fill an empty water bottle with milk. Have a friend hide the bottle somewhere in your house. Wait two weeks, then find the bottle. Open the bottle. Sniff.

Do this several times so you can build up a tolerance for the numerous wretched bottles you will lose and then unfortunately find over the course of your child's babyhood.

14

AND NOW, WE NEST

Or not

S INCE THE BEGINNING of time, pregnant women have been overcome by a primal urge to prepare their home for their unborn child. They have cleaned and painted and organized and assembled. They have made DIY mobiles and baby-proofed every cupboard in sight.

This need comes from somewhere deep inside of a pregnant woman, a switch that is flipped alerting the rest of the body that it's go time for motherhood.

This phase has come to be known as *nesting*. And you've probably heard a lot about it. In fact, every time you've put a onesie away in the closet or straightened a crooked picture frame, you've probably been accused of this nesting.

"Oh, look at you, so cute, organizing the fridge. It's the nesting instinct, you know."

To which you might have answered, "Well, I'm just putting the food away that I bought at the store. I'm not sure what my pregnancy has to do with it."

To which there was probably the response of a knowing nod, because of course you were nesting and had no idea.

The nesting instinct can be very, very strong for some women, whereas others couldn't possibly be bothered to exert the amount of energy needed to get into it. There is no way to tell where you are going to land on the scale, but I say lean into whatever nesting instincts you have, no matter how little or big they are.

The months before your baby arrives will be the last time you are able to get anything done around your house for a very long time, so it's probably a good idea to take advantage of it. It's not that you won't ever be able to accomplish another house project after you have a baby, but let's just say your schedule isn't going to be quite as open post-birth. Finding the time to hang pictures or paint a wall will fall very far down on your "Shit I Have Energy For" list once you are a parent. (At the top of the list will be "Staring at my ugly walls for five minutes without blinking, because I think I might have just fallen asleep while sitting up." [It's a really fun list.])

If you are overcome with the need to orchestrate a deep cleaning on your house, or to reorganize every cupboard at 10 PM, go for it. Warn your partner to stay out of your way, though, because you cannot and will not be stopped. It's best for everyone if you are allowed your time in your nesting spiral.

If you aren't feeling a nesting instinct, that's okay too. But do yourself a favor and at least get some important stuff done. Get a crib, or at least a bassinet, and a comfy chair for feedings. You don't have to paint or go overboard with decor, but you'll thank yourself later if you organize the clothes by size and set up a stack of diapers or two. Do it for Future Tired You.

If you really want to do Future Tired You a favor, you also might want to stock up on quick and easy meals, like canned soups, dinners from the frozen-food aisle, and peanut butter and jelly (peanut butter and jelly is going to make a big reappearance in your life soon enough anyway, and you'll realize how much you've missed it the last 15 years or so). You could also prepare some meals and freeze them in advance. Or, if your cooking abilities are in line with mine, you can find out what restaurants around you offer delivery services. Grab their menus and make a little binder for easy perusing. Future Tired You loves delivery.

Moms on the Front Lines

TO NEST OR NOT

When I asked my MOFL about their nesting instinct, they seemed to range from OCD to "Oh, is there a baby coming soon?"

SARAH: "I cleaned and reorganized the entire house. I painted the nursery, which took over 20 hours because I painted polka dots on the lower half of the wall."

DEBBIE: "We moved when I was pregnant. This may come as a surprise to you but I retiled the boy's entire bathroom floor at 8.5 months pregnant. That was just one room . . . it got much worse."

TARA: "We moved into a new house and I wasn't able to do a lot of it myself. I mostly just bossed my husband and our parents around."

MICHELLE: "I was working full time and figured I would nest once I was on maternity leave. I had exactly seven days off work before I had my son two and a half weeks early! Who does that with their first?! I was too busy visiting with family, napping, and getting ready for Christmas to deal with any nesting."

MELANIE: "Nesting, what is that!?! I was at work one day, my water broke overnight, I was in the hospital the next day, and the following day he arrived. Three weeks early. The only thing I had done to prepare was pack my husband a bag of treats for the hospital stay. That was handy."

STEPHANY: "I did not nest! I think I was worried to do too much for fear it'd jinx the pregnancy . . . or maybe I was really lazy! We didn't even pick our crib up from the store until he was over six months old. In my defense, I thought I'd have more time since he was my first. He was a week early. For some reason, I was absolutely certain he'd be late."

Stephany made the common assumption that her first baby would be late. It's an old wives' tale we all hear, and for some reason it sticks.

We did something similar but instead of assuming Vivian would be late, we looked at the due date as an absolute arrival date. As though we were picking up the child at the airport. "She is due on the 23rd, so we still have a few weeks."

Becky had major house projects planned for the week before Vivian was due, and she immediately started doing some of them when I went into labor a week early. Because installing a ceiling fan is a perfectly logical way to pass the time when someone is having contractions in the next room.

Don't be like us. Get your shit together before you are having contractions. Get a crib or a bassinet, buy some diapers, and organize the closet a bit. You might be a procrastinator, but there's no guaranteeing that your baby is inheriting that trait.

Dear Bean Letters
Week 35, Nesting

Dear Bean,

Today we finally got around to ordering your nursery furniture. This is great news, as generally it's a good idea to have a nursery set up in advance of a baby coming to live in your home. At least this is what I've been told.

Apparently, because I am pregnant, I am supposed to be very interested in getting this house ready for you. There is supposed to be a hormone swirling around my body that inspires me to nest. Unfortunately for you, I think I'm nesting-deficient. I mean, I understand on a logical level that it's important to get the house ready for your arrival. But on an emotional level I'm not quite ready to dive in.

And there will need to be diving. Because the amount of crap we have piled up in your nursery has become a bit daunting. For the past seven months or so we have been accumulating any and all things baby. We've gladly taken boxes and boxes of hand-me-downs, friends and family have bought you piles of gifts, and we've had three (THREE) baby showers. I guess gathering all of this stuff is a sort of nesting, in that we are gathering up everything we need to build the nest.

The problem is, all of this baby stuff amounts to the twigs and leaves of our nest. And instead of spending time assembling the nest, we have just thrown all the twigs and leaves (and burp cloths) into your room and quickly shut the door behind them. We've been throwing/shutting for months now and the floor of your room is officially a distant memory. There are boxes on boxes, bags on bags, and nothing on furniture, because we don't have any of that yet. But we do have some really nice twigs and leaves in that pile, so at least our nest has a lot of potential.

When we ordered your crib and dresser today, the saleslady said it would arrive in four to six weeks. I shrugged and said okay. It wasn't until later that I realized that you are due in five weeks and may beat your bed home.

It's not that we aren't excited for you to arrive, for you to need all of the stuff currently jammed into your room. But it still seems absolutely surreal that you are planning an appearance in a few short weeks. I've spent years dreaming about you, and now that you are so close to being real I'm having a little trouble believing it.

It took me months to work up the courage to actually buy you anything from the baby store. Because somehow it felt like bragging. "Look at me! I'm having a baby! She will be perfect and healthy and of course I will get to use all of this baby stuff I'm buying because my pregnancy is destined for greatness!" I wasn't comfortable bragging so early on in my pregnancy. What if something went wrong?

Even now I feel like setting up your nursery could jinx this thing we have going. Painting walls, sorting clothes, and coordinating bedding feels cocky. Something could still go wrong.

But I'm 35 weeks pregnant. You spend your days (and mostly my nights) flipping and kicking and generally keeping me very aware that you are very real. It's officially time to stop worrying about all *the things that could go wrong. And to start decorating for all the things that are going to go right.*

So tomorrow we will throw open the door to your room, wade into our twigs and leaves, and start assembling your nest. We will organize your clothes by size, we will pile diapers and bibs and burp cloths in an orderly fashion, we will assemble baby whatnots with abandon.

And slowly we will find that floor that has been lost to my fear for so many months.

It's a really nice floor. Which is good, because you may be sleeping on it until your crib arrives.

TRY NOT TO THINK ABOUT THE CHILDBIRTH MATH TOO MUCH

15

Maybe concentrate more on the possibility of an epidural

I'M A PLANNER. I like to be prepared. I like to be good at things. Although I'm creative, I also thrive on order, routine, and logic. Once I find a solution to a problem, I like using that solution over and over again to make my life easier.

This way of tackling obstacles has come in very handy throughout my life.

But it is absolute shit when applied to anything having to do with pregnancy, children, and parenting in general.

Before they even arrive, babies have a way of letting it be known that they have no time for any attempts at order and/or logic. Pregnancy will become the first in a never-ending string of child-related equations that seem to mock you with their frustrating inability to be solved.

Most frustratingly immune to all attempts at research and planning is *Baby Day One: The Delivery*.

Sure, pregnancy is pretty predictable. There are doctors and books and apps that can tell you what is happening to and inside your body at every second of the 40-week science experiment your uterus is conducting. But no matter how many doctors, books, and apps you consult, none can tell you with absolute certainty how that science experiment is going to make its way out of said uterus.

It's actually quite appropriate that you begin this parenting adventure with feelings of confusion and incompetence, as you try to wrap your brain around the imminent exit of a watermelon from your decidedly less-than-watermelon-size escape route. Confusion and incompetence are going to become pretty standard throughout this journey, so you might as well get comfortable with them early on.

There's just so much you can't know for sure. Will you have a natural birth? A cesarean? Will the baby come early or late or right on time? Will it come quickly or take its sweet time making an appearance? And most important, will you poop on the table during delivery?

All those books and doctors and apps tend to do a collective shoulder shrug when asked to give expectant moms a firm answer to the age-old question, "How will this child make its way out of me?"

Sure, you can make a birth plan. You can spend nine months outlining every detail of your vision, down to the music that will be playing and the lighting in the delivery room. You can color code this plan. You can put "My Birth Plan" at the top of the page in a modern yet sophisticated font. You can print multiple copies, laminate them (because things can get messy and you are prepared for such things), and hand them out to all the potential players (no, it doesn't hurt to give a copy to your favorite taxi driver, you never know if his services will be required). And if doing all that helps ease your mind, then by all means, laminate away.

But when it comes to *Baby Day One: The Delivery,* it's best for you to accept early and often that no amount of research or lamination or color coding is going to change the fact that you really have no idea how everything is going to go down.

I don't mean for this to freak you out even more than you are already freaked out about your delivery. My hope is to actually help you relax a bit and let go of some of the stress that comes with trying to orchestrate a situation that is so far beyond your ability to control.

The first time I was pregnant, I obsessed over how the delivery would play out. I read birth stories, I watched birth videos, I went to birthing classes. I asked my poor doctor hundreds of questions about every possible birthing scenario. Which were the best? Which were the worst? How bad can it get? What's the craziest thing she'd ever seen? I gathered all this information under the guise of educating myself. Because the more I knew, the less surprises there could be, right?

But really I was just obsessing over something I had very little control over. And no matter how much information I gathered, my birth story was going to unfold however it decided to.

I tried to remind myself of this fact often, even as I was stockpiling any and all birthing possibilities. I worked to maintain a pretty go-with-the-flow attitude about my impending birth. I didn't craft a multi-page birth plan. I was chill, I was Zen, I was prepared to take things as they came.

I mean, as long as they came with drugs. Obviously.

Epidural, epidural, and a side of epidural were the only things I knew for sure I needed during my delivery. The shining promise of an epidural was the one thing that kept my brain from overloading while contemplating the childbirth math. Delivering a baby was scary as hell, but I could totally do it. As long as I was guaranteed to not actually have to feel any of it, of course. You didn't really expect me to be Zen without pharmaceutical intervention, did you?

My biggest fear was that I would arrive at the hospital too late to get that fantasized-over epidural. But I also didn't want to arrive so early that they sent me home for being a big wimp who thought she was ready to push when she was only one centimeter dilated.

The good news is, it turns out I'm not a wimp. The bad news is my biggest fear occurred after I was wheeled into the hospital screaming for drugs and was denied them because I was 9.5 centimeters dilated by the time I got there. This was very bad news. And was also the end of the Zen, coincidently.

I go into great detail about my first delivery in my book *The Sh!t No One Tells You: A Guide to Surviving Your Baby's First Year*, should you be looking for a play-by-play on that particular birth story. But I will sum it up for you here:

- Arrive at hospital
- Scream for drugs
- Denied drugs
- Many many f-words
- Sliced whooha
- Baby pops out less than an hour after arriving at hospital
- The End

Why am I not going into great detail about my delivery in a book titled *The Sh!t No One Tells You About Pregnancy?*

Because I personally think people tell you too much shit about the birth process. The universe apparently has some unwritten rule wherein a woman must be bombarded with any and all birth stories the second she is noticeably pregnant.

"You know, my sister's friend's cousin had the craziest thing happen during her delivery!"

"Oh, please do tell me all about it, because I wasn't really wanting to have a peaceful slumber tonight anyway."

I'm not going to tell you the finer details of either of my births (the second one involved wonderful, wonderful drugs and took hours upon hours to play out) because I don't think my births have anything to do with your birth, and neither birth story involves me saying, "Dude, the baby *fell out*. No lie, like she was greased up or something. Easiest thing I've ever done." And unless I'm able to offer you that sort of reassurance, I don't want to contribute to your anxiety.

I asked my MOFL whether they felt the same way about hearing birth stories while pregnant, and their opinions were mixed.

Sarah, mom of two, said she loved hearing birth stories: "But then I would stay awake all night worrying about the actual birth!"

Jen didn't mind hearing different stories, unless they contained tales of tearing or pooping: "I was mortified of pooping happening during childbirth. So the whole time I pushed during Austin's birth I kept repeating, 'I'm so sorry if I poop.' Over and over. Poor nurses."

Brooke, who was not meaning to, actually made my point with her opinion: "I liked hearing stories! But each individual birth goes how it goes. Hearing stories doesn't change that."

Yes! It goes how it goes. And it's going to go whether you spend your pregnancy gathering piles of information or you pass the time binge watching *Breaking Bad* (and watching a show about a peaceful man who transforms into a ruthless drug lord might actually give you some ideas on how to handle the situation if you too are denied an epidural during your delivery). Delivering a baby isn't a test that you will fail if you don't study enough. And you aren't going to be sent home from the hospital in the middle of your birth and told to return when you've perfected your Lamaze breathing.

When that baby decides it's time (or your doctor decides it's time), your birth will unfold in whatever way it's going to. Getting too wrapped up in how it's going to unfold is a good way to experience a nine-month panic attack, followed by a delivery filled with an extraordinary amount of f-bombs (not that there is anything wrong with f-bombs as a relaxation technique).

Jen learned this lesson with her first delivery, after spending months diligently preparing and planning for her birth. "I think I read every book on what to expect. I took two different classes. I had a detailed birth plan! I was *well* prepared. Then when it came time to actually birth the baby, all that shit went out the window and I just started screaming, 'GIVE ME DRUGS NOW!'"

Another MOFL, Mary, was an encyclopedia of birthing knowledge when she went into her first delivery. She even took hypnobirthing classes to help her with her Zen. Then her birth plan went a little off the rails. "Man, I studied birth like it was my job! I was an idiot. It set me up with high expectations (peaceful home birth, no drugs, relaxed with no pain). And when it all went to shit, I had a really hard time getting over it. I think the hypnobirthing classes were good for the deep breathing aspect. Laboring at home was helped by that for a little while. Seventeen hours later, I was screaming in a hospital like everyone else! The second time was much better. I went the doctor/hospital route and just let it all go. Much easier, less PTSD!"

My recommendations for preparing for your birth? Plug your ears when anyone starts to tell you a birth story. Odds are they aren't anxious to tell you a story that isn't in some way bat-shit crazy.

Another recommendation: Don't Google anything having to do with delivery complications. Just don't. Your doctors and nurses and midwives have already Googled everything and, you know, even spent decades actually studying the medicine having to do with the delivering of babies. It's almost as if it's their job.

Also, don't Google the word *episiotomy*. More nope.

More advice: Accept that when a human pushes hard enough to get another human out of her body that same human is also pushing hard enough to get poop out of her body. It's just a fact. It'll probably happen. I know it sounds horrifying, but let me calm your fears by assuring you that you will have no idea that it is happening, nor will it seem like that big of a deal compared to the human body pushing its way out of you at the time. And also, those doctors and nurses deliver babies all day, you are not the first person (that hour) who has pooped in front of them.

I also recommend avoiding the birthing classes if at all possible, because they are a day-long freak-out fest. They will show you videos, give you tips, and distribute pamphlets. But somehow they leave you feeling less prepared than when you entered the room.

I retained two things from my birthing class:

1. Sitting on a yoga ball will "help" when dealing with contractions.
This was bullshit and didn't help at all because it turns out nothing helps the feeling of a human trying to force its way out of your vagina.

2. A partner can "assist" the birthing Baby Mama by offering her ice chips and/or Chapstick.
The Chapstick one really struck us as particularly funny, because it seemed so absurd to think that Chapstick would in any way assist in the delivering of a human baby. In the weeks leading up to the birth Becky would constantly offer me Chapstick when I complained about whatever pregnancy discomfort I was experiencing at the moment. We'd laaaaugh. Then she offered it on our drive to the hospital, in an attempt to distract me from my excruciating pain. I told her to shut the hell up.

Seriously. Skip the birthing class and spend the day getting a couple's massage and/or doing something you enjoy doing together that won't be possible once there is a baby added to your equation. (Might I suggest binge watching *Breaking Bad*?)

YOUR BIRTH STORY will be nothing like any that you've ever heard, because none of those stories involved your negotiating a person out of your own uterus. There's no book or blog you can read that will tell you about your birth story, because your story hasn't been written yet. When it is written it will seem similar to other stories, yet somehow magnificently unique. Just like the baby it brings into the world.

Birth is just a tiny blimp in the scheme of pregnancy and parenting, a matter of hours out of a whole lifetime. You can do anything for a matter of hours, especially if you know there is a new baby waiting for you at the end.

So, instead of frantically researching all the different ways a delivery can go, why don't you Google adorable newborn photos, because I guarantee they are the best part of any birth story. And those pictures are the beautiful ending you should be keeping in mind no matter what happens during your story.

Or maybe watch some of those videos that play before an athlete competes in the Olympics. The ones that show all the work they put in, all the sacrifices, pulled muscles, setbacks, and sweat that led to their big gold-medal moment.

Your road to your baby, however winding or difficult, is almost to its gold-medal end. You just have to get through the last 50-yard dash of childbirth. Or maybe I should compare childbirth to curling, because no one has any idea what is going on in curling. There are a lot of people working very hard, frantic, frowning, and yelling, all trying to get the curling thing to the middle of a bull's-eye. There are hugs and high fives when the bull's-eye is hit. Just like childbirth.

So take a deep breath and get Zen about what is coming your way. The end of pregnancy, the beginning of your baby, and the best gold medal anyone has ever received.

Partner Corner

If you've read the rest of this chapter, you will see that I highly recommend that your Baby Mama go into her delivery with a laid-back approach. I've told her that the doctors and nurses have it handled. That everything is going to be fine. And it probably will. But it also might not.

And that's where you come in, dear partner.

You have a job during the delivery and it is nearly as important as the job the Baby Mama has, because it's your job to keep the Baby Mama from losing her shit during labor. Or, if she's losing her shit, then at the very least you need to try to keep her from going completely off the rails.

And while I tried to discourage your Baby Mama from getting too wrapped up in planning an unplannable birthing experience, I'm going to need you to get your plan on well before go time.

Now, you don't need to make a four-page birth plan or even watch a lot of birthing videos to prepare, but you do need to ask some questions. Your Baby Mama most likely has some ideas of how she wants her birth to go down. And you probably think she'll do just fine letting those ideas be known, because you've never known her to be particularly shy when asked to express an opinion.

But here's the thing. She's going to have a person pushing its way out of her. So she might not be in the right frame of mind to articulate her thoughts. And at the time her thoughts will primarily be made up of loud screeching sounds and regret for thinking any of this was a good idea.

➤

That's where you come in.

Yes, there will be highly skilled nurses and doctors and more nurses and doctors. But your Baby Mama is going to need you to be her voice to those nurses and doctors, if her voice is preoccupied with screaming the before mentioned f-bombs.

BEFORE THE BIRTH

A few months before the baby is due, sit down with your Baby Mama and hash out some details:

- Does she want drugs?
- Does she want a doula?
- Does she want to be induced?
- Does she want a C-section?
- Does she want skin to skin contact right after the baby is born?
- Who does she want in the room with her when the baby is being born?
- Does she want any special music/outfit/birthing ball?
- Is there anything else that is especially important to her? Anything she is especially scared of?

Talk about all of these things, write down her answers. Talk about them again as the due date gets closer. Study them. You will be tested later.

DURING THE BIRTH

Your job is to take all of her wishes with you into that delivery room and to fight for them if she needs you to. Your job is also to not fight too hard if at any point she says she's changed her mind.

I didn't say your job was easy.

If you are confused about whether you should fight for something or give in, ask the doctors and nurses to give you a few minutes alone to discuss the issue. Once you are alone, take a deep breath, ask her what she wants, and then try to make that happen for her. If you can't make it happen, try to calm her fears and assure her everything is going to be okay, even if you don't know that.

AFTER THE BIRTH

After the baby arrives, you are still on the job. Now your job is doubled. Your Baby Mama may be tired or sore or overwhelmed, so she still needs your help. And your baby, well, it's a baby, so it's going to need your help for a while.

If your Baby Mama is planning on nursing, ask for a lactation consultant as soon as that baby pops out, and pay attention when that consultant visits. Keep taking your notes. You are getting so much extra credit, I promise.

After both of our kids were born, my partner stayed with them wherever they went. She held their hands as they were being cleaned up, she went with them when they had to get any testing done, she stood watch when the nurses poked and prodded. She was my eyes and ears, which allowed me to relax a little, knowing that they were being protected.

You may have no idea what to do with a birthing Baby Mama or a newborn, but that's okay. Just show up, be prepared to speak up, and watch over both of them. Be a real partner.

Also, you too are entitled to liberal use of f-bombs, which you will most likely find quite helpful while navigating this time (and for the next few years, to be honest).

Go, team!

Partner Corner

BRINGING OUT BABY

JEREMY: "As the D-day neared, the anxiety built (first time around anyway). But I was never 'scared' until there was a real chance (I mean a genuine fucking chance) I was gonna lose both of them during labor with the first kid, and there wasn't a damn thing I could do about it. I was helpless. I'm the guy who fixes things, everything. I can build hotrods from scratch, I design thousands of complete vehicles at work and get them built. But in that case I didn't have the tools, and that sucked."

KRISTA: "The experience of being on what's typically a male side of the birth experience was amazing. I saw the experience of birth in a whole new way. I watched the miracle of it and cut the cord. I felt at such a loss as to how to help my wife handle the pain, but I was mesmerized by the birth of my third son."

JASON: "We had our second son at home. It was the most relaxing thing ever. No stress at all. We even visited the Jack in the Box drive-thru to get her a shake about six hours into labor. I just let her do what she wanted to do and we had a very relaxing time. I know it sounds odd."

MATT: "My wife was in labor and I kept saying, 'C'mon! Time to go!'

"She stopped, looked at me and said, 'Um. I'm not going anywhere.' What?! 'Grab some towels.' I need to wash my hands! 'You don't have time.' What?! 'He's coming!' I threw towels on the ground, called 911, and Griffin's head came out.

"Birthing Griffin in the hallway has given us a special bond. I don't believe in baloney like drinking warm water before bed to melt fat or that kale is good for you, but I do believe that Griffin and I have a special daddy/son relationship. Maybe it's because he's the youngest and he's so damn cute. Or maybe it's because he dropped into my arms while I had the phone between my ear and shoulder, screaming at the 911 operator who was trying to help me birth this kid. Meanwhile imaginary block text was streaming across my field of vision, 'THIS IS NOT HAPPENING.'

"But it happened. We all survived. I was so amped, I beat the ambulance to the hospital (with my wife and son in it)."

Your Pregnancy Week by Week

HOW BIG IS YOUR BABY?

WEEKS 35–37—TRY NOT TO THINK ABOUT IT

These are the weeks when we start running out of items in the produce section that are big enough to accurately be compared to your growing fetus. We are now forced to head over to the bulk aisle for adequate comparisons. Or, better yet, let's head to the pet store.

Your baby is between 18 and 19 inches during these weeks and I think it's a lot easier to imagine him or her as a tiny animal (such as a puppy or a soft rabbit) instead of a very large piece of fruit. Animals are cute and snuggly and a lot more visually appealing than a melon of any sort.

So, instead of visualizing cold hard melons, let's think about hugging a golden retriever puppy. You just can't go wrong with visualizing a puppy.

Pregnancy WOD
MONTH 9

If you have ever trained for a long-distance run like a full or a half-marathon then you are likely familiar with "recovery days" and the tapering that comes at the end of your training. You spend months pushing your body and gradually increasing your mileage, and then in the few weeks before the big event, you taper off to allow your body a little recovery time before tackling your final run.

Parenting is a lot like a marathon, if a marathon lasted for decades instead of a few hours. So I have designed my training program in a similar fashion to a marathon training program. This last month, we are all about tapering. And by "tapering" I mean "napping." Because, of course.

1. Nap for as long as your body will allow. Then nap a little more.

16

GOOD NEWS: YOU'RE EATING FOR TWO. BAD NEWS: BOTH OF YOU REALLY LIKE ICE CREAM

Mumus might be your only option from here on out

*A*T THIS POINT in your pregnancy, you may officially be all out of shits. You are in the homestretch, you can almost taste the epidural (it tastes like sunshine and poppy fields, FYI), and you don't particularly care that you look like you are carrying a litter of children in your uterus. You are big and beautiful, or at least big and all out of shits.

Pregnancy weight gain can vary for every women. Some women balloon up to a size that seems almost mathematically impossible, and others barely look pregnant until you see them from the side and notice their cute little belly. Sometimes women can spend most of their pregnancy in the "cute belly" category and then all of a sudden hurdle over into the "balloon" category in the final few weeks. I'm not sure if there is a scientific reason for this last minute expansion, but I think it might have something to do with carbohydrates.

In these last few weeks you should heed the advice of your doctor if he or she seems concerned about your weight. But if your doctor doesn't seem concerned? It's officially F-it time.

Eat whatever you want, reward your hard work, and enjoy these last few weeks of guilt-free calorie consumption.

When I was 40 weeks pregnant, we visited a restaurant that was offering deep-fried cheesecake with a side of ice cream, whipped cream, and raspberry sauce. I ordered it as my main course. Because F-it.

You may be too tired or sore or lazy to move much these last few weeks. F-it. You know what doesn't take any energy? Eating ice cream and binge-watching trashy television shows. Do that. All of that. Fall asleep doing that. Because nothing says 40 weeks pregnant like waking up at 2 PM covered in melted ice cream. You are a champion.

As soon as that baby pops out, you will feel pressure (mostly self-imposed) to take off all this baby weight (it's nice that they call it "baby" weight instead of "ice cream and Netflix" weight, which is what it actually is). But let's save that stress for a later date. We have enough stress right now. Because we have opened a family-size bag of chips and we can't find a chip clip, and the only way to keep the chips from going stale is to eat the whole bag. It's a very trying time.

My point is, you are a badass who has grown a person inside of your body. This has not been easy. And we won't even get into how much more badassery is going to be needed to get the person *out* of your body. You deserve to treat yourself a little bit. I would tell you to do anything that makes you happy right now, but you are uncomfortable and irritable and very big. So your happy options are limited. Which leaves calorie intake as one of your few reliable routes to smiles.

So F-it. And eat it.

Moms on the Front Lines

I asked my MOFL about their pregnancy weight gain and if the increasing scale number traumatized them. I also wanted to know whether they were able to take off the weight following their delivery and how their bodies looked post-baby-making. None of us seemed to have made it out unscathed.

SOMMER: "I gained 45 pounds. And I only lost six in the delivery. Everyone said that I would feel so thin after delivery. No, I did not!! It took a good year to get off the rest. With working out, running small races, hiring a personal trainer, and eating healthy. Apparently my body wanted to stay fat a little bit longer."

JEN: "I gained, like, 60 pounds with my first. I stopped working out when I found out I was pregnant because I was so nervous (first child syndrome). Towards the end I literally stopped caring at all and I was eating an Oreo cookie milk shake every single night. I lost all the weight and then some. When I was pregnant with my second, I was doing Boot Camp five days a week. Racing and frog leaps up until I was six months pregnant. I barely gained any weight. Then I was put on partial bedrest because my cervix was soft (I'm guessing it could have been the frog leaps; just saying). That's when I started putting on weight."

DANA: "I was totally traumatized by the weight gain with my first pregnancy because over half of it was put on in the first half of the pregnancy. I think by 20 weeks I had gained 10 pounds between monthly appointments. My doctor told me to slow down. I had no idea why it was happening so fast, but I did eat a lot of ice cream. I left the hospital both times having only lost what my baby weighed. I did get it all off over the course of a year both times with diet, exercising, and nursing. However, my body, even at my pre-pregnancy weight, does NOT look the same."

TARA: "I worked out throughout almost all of my first pregnancy. With my second I gave up almost immediately. I just didn't have it in me. I don't have a weight issue now, but my stomach looks like a popped balloon and the rest of me will never be the same. Time to bury the bikini and go shopping for a cover-up."

Partner Corner
BIG AND BEAUTIFUL

MATT: "It was neat, seeing her grow . . . And grow . . . And grow. She had a crazy appetite. Pickles at midnight were nothing. Try kimchi at 3 AM! Or peanut butter pickle toast with ice chips that only came from a corner bakery five cities away."

BECKY: "She didn't get huge. She was adorable."

JEREMY: "I had no problem with her getting bigger; she was cute."

KEVIN: "I think women are beautiful when they're pregnant. My wife is very beautiful, and in my mind, that only intensified with her pregnancy."

JASON: "With the first pregnancy she gained 80 pounds and had complications because of it. I got her into eating healthy and juicing to better combat the issues she was having and I worked to support her when she was having a tough day. All I could do was try my best to be there for her and take a lot of photos of her to assure her that she was still beautiful."

Partner Corner

ADVICE FOR
SURVIVING PREGNANCY

JASON: "Let her cry and don't always try to fix it; she doesn't want it fixed, she just wants to know you care."

JEREMY: "Relax . . . it will all be fine. And also, maybe grab some booze."

KEVIN: "Always be present for your wife, ESPECIALLY when she's pregnant. I don't just mean be in the room with her: Actually be there—both in mind and body."

MATT: "Don't run away. Don't give up. It will be okay. Sleep is overrated anyway, and you can catch up on your rest when they're older. Keep the compliments up and keep doing 110 percent, whether or not you feel like it. It's time to grow up, and growing up is okay. It's all worth it."

Your Pregnancy Week by Week

HOW BIG IS YOUR BABY?

WEEKS 38–40

At this point, you are about full term. You know what size your baby is? It's about the size of, wait for it . . . a baby. Yes, we have officially moved beyond the theoretical and into reality. The reality is, you have a full-size baby in your uterus as we speak (or read). And while that's scary, it's also really exciting, I swear! You're almost there!

If you are wondering how big a newborn baby is, there are ways to gather this information. You could seek out a person who owns a new baby, or maybe look up a picture of a newborn on the Internet. But honestly, at this point, I'd caution against any of that. What good could come of it, really? You'd find a baby, you'd hold it, you'd look at the size of its head, you'd start visualizing your own impending birth, and then you'd have a three-week panic attack.

These are your last weeks of freedom. Instead of breathing heavily into a paper bag, you should be napping and eating ice cream sundaes (in whatever order you choose).

So put your pregnancy app down, walk away, and think tiny, soft thoughts. Do it for your brain. Do it for your vagina. She has enough stress coming her way; let her have a little time off.

17

PACKING FOR THE HOSPITAL

Don't overthink it

$\mathcal{M}$ ANY WOMEN HOPE that their attention to packing predelivery will somehow positively influence the ease of their birth. If they pack just the right combo of items into their Going to the Hospital Bag, perhaps everything else will fall into place and their delivery will go off without a hitch! They spend months creating the perfect list of bringable items, rounding up each object, and arranging them in their bag with Tetris-like precision.

Other women are like me and wake up one morning with contractions and tell their partner it might be a good idea to pack a bag. When that partner asks what to pack, these women shrug, and then their partners shove roughly 872 items that happen to be in the general vicinity of their packing frenzy into a plastic bag from Target.

If you are in the Tetris category, there's not much I can do to advise you on bag strategy. Because I'm assuming you've already purchase three other books on the topic. And if packing 362 items helps you maintain your Zen before your due date, then pack away. You most likely won't actually use 359 of the items in your bag, but being overly prepared may provide you a certain amount of reassurance as you head into childbirth. And anything that reassures is fine by me.

If you are in the shrug category, I'm probably not going to motivate you to change your personality type. The thought of packing a bag might stress you out, or annoy you, and I don't want to be responsible for either of those emotions in a pregnant lady.

But I will tell you that you don't need a whole lot at the hospital, and the more you bring, the more you have to lug around from room to room throughout your stay. If you forget something, you can always send your partner out to get a needed item, or ask a friend to bring it for you.

Here are a few things I think are worth throwing in a bag:

Comfy, Loose Clothing, Such as a Swimsuit Cover

The gowns they provide at the hospital are less than dignified, and often leave you flashing your ass to the whole world every time you get up to pee. If you would like to spare the whole world this treat, you can grab a couple of soft swimsuit covers to wear during your birth and after. The ones I brought were strapless, fit snug around my boobs, and were loose down to my mid-thigh. They were very comfortable, allowed for easy access to my boobs and nether regions (two hotspots during delivery and your hospital stay) and still let me feel covered up.

Toiletries

A nice shower will be ever so lovely after giving birth, so pack your favorite soap, shampoo, and conditioner to help you start feeling a little normal. Also, don't forget your toothbrush and toothpaste.

Snacks

For you. For your partner. For the labor. For post-baby. You can never go wrong having snacks at arm's reach.

Loose, Disposable Underwear

The hospital will have amazing mesh underwear for you to wear after birth, but you might want your own. Don't bring anything you are too attached to, because it most likely won't survive what is coming out of your body.

Nursing Tank Top

If you plan to nurse, you might want to bring a nursing tank top. I had a few of these and I wore them around the clock for about a year after both of my kids were born. Because I'm all about fashion.

These things are like regular nursing bras, which offer you the ability to pop a boob out at any time, but they are built into a tank top that covers your belly. They are delightful.

Outfits for the Baby

Throw a bunch of onesies in the bag for the baby, because they will soil through a few a day at least. Otherwise your baby will be stuck wearing hospital onesies, which are about as pleasant as any other institutional wear. Look for onesies that have wide necks or zippers and not tons of buttons, because life it too short to spend it buttoning buttons that will only have to be unbuttoned four minutes later.

Also, bring that one special "Going Home" outfit for the baby. And maybe one for you too. Think loose and comfy for your outfit, adorable and picture-worthy for the child.

Another Bag

Bring along another empty bag. This is key. You know when you go on vacation and sometimes you bring an extra bag to hold all the crap you are going to buy on vacation? This is kind of like that, except instead of tacky magnets you are going to want to bring home a ton of industrial-size maxi pads. And those things take up a lot of room.

The hospital will have all sorts of things worth taking home, and you don't want to be left without a proper transportation device. First and foremost, you need to grab as many of the hospital nose-sucker things as you can get your hands on. Start on day one and take all the replacement ones they bring in to restock your room. For some reason the nose-sucker things from the hospital are the only nose-sucker things that actually work. Grab 300. Also grab diapers, hats, blankets, ladybit numbing spray, and perhaps a nurse or two. Bring a bag big enough to take them all home with you.

Treats for the Nurses

This isn't required, but it's a nice thing to do. Nurses help you around the clock during your delivery and your first hours/days following your child's birth. They are attentive, informed, and answer all your stupid questions as if they haven't heard them 395 times (that day). Bring them a box of chocolate or some other treat to show that you appreciate what they do every day for new babies and new parents. Also, maybe if you bribe them with sweets, they will look the other way when you leave the hospital with $36,000 in baby items in your extra bag.

DON'T WORRY ABOUT packing diapers; the hospital will have plenty for you. And, of course, pack anything else that you feel may help you through the process of birthing and caring for a newborn baby (a nanny, perhaps?). But just know that your hospital is in the business of taking care of moms in labor and newborn babies, so they might be fully stocked up on everything you will need.

Except the nanny, unfortunately.

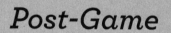

Post-Game

18

THEY WILL LET YOU TAKE A NEWBORN BABY HOME

Yes, that's scary as hell

I HAVE SOME NEWS for you. You might want to sit down for this one. It's going to blow your mind.

After you have a baby and the doctors determine that it is healthy, you will be allowed to take that baby home. With you. In a car.

You will not be made to pass any tests or run through any obstacle courses. They will not ask you for letters of recommendation or references to call. They will not hand you any sort of instruction manual, nor will they confirm that you've done any independent research into caring for a child. They won't check that your car seat is installed correctly or do a home visit to make sure you are taking the baby to a safe environment.

They will just let you leave the hospital, carrying a baby. I think they require you to name the child and sign discharge papers, but other than that, you are free to go!

This was and remains absolutely mind-boggling to me. I had to jump through more hoops when adopting my cat than when I took home my babies. When you leave the hospital and get to your car, you may find yourself looking around, checking to see whether anyone is running after you. Because, obviously, it can't be this easy to take off with a child. I mean, they are aware that you are completely unqualified for this job, right? And that this job is probably the most important one on the planet? Anyone? Hello?

One of my MOFL, Sarah, is a veterinarian, and was very alarmed when she left the hospital with her first child: "We actually stopped when we got out of the hospital. We looked around and thought, are they actually letting us leave with him?! I mean, I give more detailed written instructions when I send a dog home after being spayed!!"

So brace yourselves, dear readers, because you too will be shocked when you are allowed to leave the hospital with your baby. Try not to look too shocked, though, because that might make people suspicious.

There is little that you can do to magically make yourself confident in your parenting abilities, but you can at least set yourself up for success. Before you go into labor, get your house stocked with piles of diapers, burp cloths, swaddle blankets, baby clothes, and wipes (we used ultra-soft paper towels and warm water at the beginning; if you are going to use wipes make sure they are sensitive and alcohol-free to cut down on the chance of diaper rash). Figure out where the baby is going to be sleeping (your room or their room) and get their bed ready. Install your car seat and maybe even have it checked out by the fire station to make sure you've done it correctly. Basically, give yourself the impression that you are prepared.

Once the baby arrives, use your time in the hospital to ask as many questions as you possibly can. There are no stupid questions when it comes to trying to figure out how to care for a human child. Have the nurses show you how to do anything from swaddling to latching. Take notes (maybe on an actual piece of paper, because your brain is no longer going to be a reliable storage device) and also take as many supplies as they will allow.

When you get home with your baby, don't hesitate to call up the advice nurse with any questions or concerns. Your friends who already have children are also a great resource. Text them with abandon. Scour the Internet for opinions as well, but be warned that it is a great place to find evidence that no matter what you are doing, you are doing something wrong. So keep that in mind before you lose hours of your life to an online mom forum.

Finally, never has the phrase "Fake it till you make it" been more appropriate than when you are granted the responsibility of caring for a newborn. You know the basics. Feed them, change them, hold them, love them. Keep doing those things as if you know what you are doing, and eventually you will.

And don't worry too much; none of us knew how to parent when we left the hospital either. If they let only completely qualified people take children home, there would be roughly four million babies staying in hospitals throughout the land every year. I'm guessing that's why they aren't chasing you down the hall when you are leaving with your particular baby.

Let the wise words of my MOFL Stephany light your path as you reluctantly pull away from the hospital with your new tiny human: "When we finally left the hospital, my husband and I were crazy scared because we had no idea what to do. We had spent so much time trying to get and stay pregnant, but we had no idea what to do beyond that. I literally said to my husband as we were walking out, 'If crack addicts can keep their babies alive, we can too.' It was oddly comforting!"

So there you have it. You can do this. And the fact that you are worried about whether you can do it probably means you are going to do it just fine.

But maybe put that advice nurse on speed dial, just in case.

19

BREASTFEEDING, SLEEP TRAINING, POSTPARTUM

Your fun is just starting

𝒪N MY BOOK *The Sh!t No One Tells You: A Guide to Surviving Your Baby's First Year,* I go into quite a bit of detail about what is coming your way in the first 12 months with your child. It's a laugh a minute (the book and the year).

I was going to copy and paste the book here, but that seemed a bit excessive. Instead I've decided to focus on my top three pieces of advice for new moms. Of course, quite a few other issues will come up with your newborn, but these are the ones that I feel will get you going on the right foot.

BREASTFEEDING/BOTTLE FEEDING

Breastfeeding was by far the biggest struggle I faced when my baby was brand-new (which is saying a lot, because I was a mess). Looking back on it, I think breastfeeding was so hard because I expected it to be so easy. I expected my child to pop out, jump up to my boob, and grab on for dear life. Because her life actually depended on it. Surely nature would instill in her every instinct she needed to sustain herself. But it turns out, she didn't quite get the memo.

I had been told repeatedly throughout my pregnancy that breast was best, and that if I cared at all about my child and her future well-being, I would breastfeed. It was, of course, the most natural thing on the planet.

And then it turned out that the most natural thing on the planet took myself and two helpers to pull off at the beginning. Because sometimes nature needs an assist, apparently.

I always try to warn pregnant moms that breastfeeding will be really hard, so they go into it with that expectation. Just a tiny shift in expectation can mean the difference between sticking with it or giving up and falling into a deep depression because your body is failing at the most basic of motherly duties.

In my case, both of my kids had a sensitivity to dairy (if I drank or ate it, their bellies didn't enjoy my breast milk). I think this is a very common sensitivity and I always recommend cutting out dairy if your baby seems to be uncomfortable or gassy. It took me a week or so to figure this out with Vivian, but with Daniel I went dairy-free from the first day (in the hospital I told them I was vegan so they wouldn't give me anything with dairy). They had very different first-week experiences because of this minor change in my diet.

Also, I like to tell moms that it is not the end of the world if they aren't able to breastfeed. I know moms who chose not to, or couldn't, or tried for months and couldn't get their boobs to ever fully come on board. These moms felt shame at formula-feeding their babies, and that's not an added stress new moms need.

Whether you breastfeed or formula feed, the point is, you are feeding the child. And that is the most important part of the equation.

If you formula feed, it may take you a few tries to find a formula that your child likes (or that your child's belly likes). When trying different formulas, don't overlook the store-brand formula. They are a lot cheaper and provide the same nutrients as name brands. Also, remember that these are new bellies you are working with, so try not to change up their food too often. If you find a formula that your baby likes, stick with that one.

Basically, feeding your baby is the number one requirement for taking care of them. And it can be really demoralizing if getting them fed is difficult in any way. Try to get as much help as you can from the hospital staff before you leave. If you are breastfeeding, ask to talk to a lactation consultant two minutes after the baby arrives. Talk to them more than once.

Don't wait until things aren't working to ask for help. As with most tasks involving your baby, it's best to go into feeding assuming you know nothing. And work your way up from there.

SLEEP TRAINING

Getting your baby to sleep for extended periods of time, preferably during dark hours, will quickly become your number one parenting goal once you bring home your newborn. You will miss sleep in a way an addict misses drugs when they are forced to stop them cold turkey. Because you will essentially be stopping sleep cold turkey. And as with a drug addict, your withdrawal symptoms will not be pretty.

There is no way for you to prepare for the level of exhaustion you will feel when your baby is brand-new. And the shock it will send through your system may leave you frantically searching for a solution. But here's the thing: Babies aren't great sleepers. Some have their days and nights mixed up when they pop out; some have belly issues that make it uncomfortable to lie down; some just want to be held 24 hours a day because they are babies and they are scared.

There are countless sleep-training options out there, ranging from Cry Baby Cry to I'll Hold You Until You Are 14. I recommend investigating all of them, and trying them until you land on one that works. Stick with it as long as it works. If it stops working, go back to the drawing board.

When I brought Vivian home, I was obsessed with trying to find a sleep-training option that worked for her, because all I could think about was how long it would be until we all got to sleep like normal people again. I was so frustrated that she didn't excel at any method, and my exhaustion left me feeling defeated and sad.

But when I brought Daniel home, I knew what was coming my way. I knew I was going to be tired for a long time; I knew he wasn't going to be a perfect sleeper right out of the gate. But I didn't stress out as much with him, and even though I was still tired, I wasn't nearly as frustrated. This made a huge difference in my overall mood.

So, if you can, accept that your baby is coming into this world with the sole goal of creating permanent dark circles around your eyes. There will be nights that turn into mornings and crying that lasts what feels like three days. It's going to be hard. But I promise it's also going to be temporary.

I promise you that eventually your child will sleep, although I can't promise you that it will happen as quickly as you want it to. And I can't promise that you'll ever be allowed to sleep with the freedom and gusto that you did pre-kids.

But the first few months of exhaustion will slowly get better as your body adjusts to decreasing sleep and your child adjusts to the idea of increasing their sleep. Be patient with both of you during this time as you battle these huge learning curves. You'll both get there eventually, because there is no way a child with your DNA isn't going to be a champion sleeper someday. It's just science.

POSTPARTUM BABY BLUES

You've probably heard a lot about postpartum depression and the baby blues that can come after having a baby. But no matter how much you've heard or read, it always comes as a bit of a shock to your system when you experience it yourself.

There is something that feels inherently wrong about sadness during what should be such a happy time. You just won the lottery, dammit! Why are you crying?

But keep in mind that, yes, you just won the lottery, but then your hormones went upside down and you stopped sleeping. And the lottery check won't stop screaming. So don't beat yourself up if you are little blue. It doesn't mean you don't love your baby, and it doesn't mean you aren't up for this parenting gig. It just means you may need to break down in a heap of tears periodically for no apparent reason. Don't fight it.

Postpartum issues can range from a mild case of the baby blues all the way up to severe depression. If you are feeling sad, or overwhelmed, or just *off*, don't keep it to yourself. Share it with your partner, your doctor, and any close friends you trust. There is no shame in having postpartum sadness, and no one will fault you for it. And your lottery ticket won't love you any less, I promise.

Partner Corner
A PSA

JEREMY: "Postpartum depression was the worst because that shit is REAL and nobody ever warns you about it. Not your dad, uncle, homies . . . nobody. I swear I saw my wife's head spin around a few times. The mood swings and complete breakdowns are hard for a dude to comprehend, let alone deal with. Dudes only have one, maybe two emotions at a time, that's it. We are pretty level, predictable, reliable. Women are a strange drug for us. Unpredictable . . . bat shit crazy . . . intriguing . . . annoying . . . addictive . . .

"During the postpartum time, you expect to see somebody jump out of a bush with a camera and say, 'Ha! Gotcha!' But that moment never comes and you are left wondering, 'WTF is happening?' 'Is it permanent?' Thankfully, it's not; it all buffed out in the end. But I'm still mad that nobody warned me, and have taken it as a personal mission to PSA that shit to any dude coming close to that point in life."

Partner Corner

THOUGHTS ON THE BABY MAMA

MATT: "I'm in awe of God's thoughtful creativity. I'm in total amazement of the emotional, physical, and chemical transformation of my wife's body as she puked and grew her way through nine grueling months of hardcore body-boot-baby camp. If she'd given it up after baby #1, I would've understood. It was that tough. I think she's amazing and it's way harder than anything I could do."

KEVIN: "Men aren't shit. Women make babies."

PETE: "I remain amazed at the female body and what it can do. I watch Julie with the kids and am amazed by the woman and mother she has become. I really don't know how she does it, but I'm grateful (and need to remember to tell her that once in a while). Sometimes she complains about looking old or never losing the baby belly and it drives me crazy. Those things never bother me. In fact, they remind me of the sacrifices she has made for me—for us—for our family. I love all of it. But nothing is better than watching one of my kids and catching a glimpse of my wife in their eyes, their smile, or their mannerisms. Each one reminds me of her in different ways. I love that."

BECKY: "I loved my partner before she pushed those two watermelons out for me, but there is another layer of love that I feel because she made our kids. A kind of love that I only realize when there is enough calm to remember it. There is no one in the world that can ever replace that role for me and I am forever grateful to her and will always love her for it."

JEREMY: "Before kids, you are both selfish, and for the most part self-serving. But a strange thing happens when you have kids; there is an inherent deeper connection or bond that forms. I felt it the moment Michelle was in labor with Enzo and some pretty gnarly shit went down. At that moment, there was a very collective 'we' that formed. I had both of their backs and I was willing to do whatever it took to keep them both safe and healthy.

"At that moment, a much deeper love and appreciation of my wife formed, one that I will forever fail at accurately explaining to her. And I will continue to fall short at expressing, because I'm a dude, and we speak different languages.

"There are still fights, arguments, and disagreements . . . mostly over money and trivial things as we blindly try to make our way through life and apply all the 'filters' society says we should. But at the end of the day, from the day our first son was born till the day I die, I've got her back . . . forever."

Dear Bean Letters
Week 41 —We Made It

Dear Bean,

We made it.

We made it to the hospital before you kicked your way into the world (barely, you kicked a lot faster than I was expecting). We made it out of the hospital after having to stay an extra couple of days (turns out neither of us knew how to operate my boobs). We made it home, everyone in one piece (although my pieces are a little worse for the wear).

Since we've been home, I've found life to be a series of very loud and very quiet moments. You, my love, are responsible for both.

You are so tiny, you are swimming in your newborn onesies because they are too big for your little body. Yet you've become very good at getting your point across via a decibel that is quite ambitious for something only weighing six pounds.

Since you are so little and so new, your only form of communication is these ear-busting screams (for added fun, you are usually doing this screaming right near an actual ear). Unfortunately for all of us, I don't speak "scream" and most of the time I have no idea what you are trying to communicate exactly. Are you wet? Are you hungry? Are you tired? Are you gassy? Are you a newborn baby, and therefore you scream a lot? I just don't know.

We do a lot of holding you and bouncing you and feeding you and burping you and changing you. When you cry, we tend to do all of those things in rapid succession, hoping to land on whatever will bring you (and our ears) comfort.

And sometimes it works. You just wanted to eat, or be rocked, or be sung to, or be changed. Or maybe you just wanted to see us frantically do all those things, because we are your dancing monkeys now, and that is entertaining, even to a baby. Could go either way.

But when it works, when you are calm or when you are lulled to sleep, that's when the quiet moments take place. It is a quiet like I've never experienced (and God help anyone who makes any noise and startles you back into crying mode).

But more than just the absence of sound, these quiet moments now hold something else. You. There you are, peacefully sleeping, or peacefully eating, or just peacefully being peaceful. I stare at you during these quiet times and study you for hours. That sounds crazy, but I literally spend hours of my days just staring at you. Almost as if I need to constantly remind myself that you are actually here, that this is all real.

If you are awake I will try to talk to you a bit, but you aren't much of a conversationalist, so we usually just end up sitting in silence staring at each other. Both of us getting used to you being on the outside of me.

I most often sit with my knees up and you lying on my legs, on a little baby recliner. Your tiny feet kick, kick, kick my belly as we stare at each other. The kicking is familiar; you've been doing it to the inside of my belly for months.

You are only a couple of weeks old, but I feel like I've known you for longer than that. Because I have. And now we are like pen pals *who are meeting after years spent communicating back and forth. My communications were mostly prayers and talking to my belly, while you relied heavily on kicking and waves of nausea.*

It seems like I've dreamt of you forever, and now, here you are on my lap. Quiet, peaceful, and occasionally screaming your tiny head off.

We made it.

You're perfect.

Welcome home, Bean.

Epilogue

$\mathcal{I}$ ONCE WROTE A quote for a greeting card that read, "Pregnancy is the time in between who you were and who you were meant to be." The card had a picture of a pregnant woman looking down at her month-nine belly.

I wrote the quote before I had kids of my own. Before I realized that I was "meant to be" someone whose daily ensemble included yoga pants and dark circles under her eyes. Who knew I was meant for so much glamour?

Now that I've had pregnancies of my own, as well as the resulting babies, I've started to look at the 40 weeks of gestation a little differently. I joke throughout this book that pregnancy is crunch time. A countdown clock to parenthood. And it is. But more than that, it's a countdown to a new version of you.

Think of it as You, Version 2.0: Mom Edition.

As soon as that baby pops out, you will officially and forever be A Mom. It's big. It's amazing. It's encompassing in a way that can't really be put into words.

You will feel an overwhelming pressure to do everything you can to prepare for motherhood in the months leading up to your delivery, and all of that work and planning is valid and important. But I'd like to encourage you to do one more thing as well.

I'd like you to spend these pregnancy months taking some time to really get to know the current version of you. The woman you are today, before you forever add "Mom" to your title.

Read a bunch of novels you've had your eye on over the years. Go to the theater. Leave your phone at home and go for a walk around your neighborhood. Try out that hobby you've always been interested in. Go somewhere you've never been. Be still. Say yes if a friend invites you out. Have long, meandering conversations with your partner about nothing, and everything. Write in a journal. Get to know yourself.

Theoretically, you've had your entire life to do all these things, to learn everything you need to know about yourself, and maybe you feel adequately educated on the subject of you. Even if that's the case, go ahead and take a little refresher course.

Once you bring home your new baby (whether it's baby #1, 2, 3, or 8), your life will change forever. Because it now has to make room for a whole new person. And that new person will stake out its space splat in the middle of your home, your heart, and your mind.

There will be a haze over your life for a while, the haze that babies tend to bring along with them. You'll be tired, over-whelmed, and under-bathed. But the haze is temporary and will slowly begin to lift as your kids get a little older and you get your footing along this learning curve.

When the haze dissipates, you may wonder where you are exactly. And who you are. The truth is, you're the same person you were before that pregnancy test started you on this new path. Your heart is just a little bit bigger and your face is just a lot more in need of cosmetic help.

I want you to get to know yourself during pregnancy, because I want you to make your way back to that woman after you come out of your new-mom haze. Obviously you aren't going to make your way back to all the things you were pre-parenthood (RIP, ab muscles and relaxing Sunday afternoons doing nothing), but that doesn't mean you can't hit some of the major bullet points.

You can join a book club. Or sign up for a spin class. Or organize a moms' night out. Or take a solo stroll around your neighborhood after dinner. Or set a regular date night with your spouse.

It can be easy to lose yourself in the commotion of parenthood, but making an effort to incorporate who you were into who you are will make you better for everyone.

This is not to say that the New You isn't going to be pretty kick-ass. What New You will lack in freedom, sleep, and privacy, she will more than make up for in baby giggles, tummy time, and little hands that are always reaching out for mom, never really wanting to let her go.

As you hold on to those little hands and navigate through this new life as a mom, you'll be constantly searching for tips and tricks on how to be the best parent for your kids. I could give you piles and piles of these tips and tricks (I've filled entire books with them). But I'm not going to. I'm not going to tell you to relax (because you won't) or that it all goes by so fast (because it doesn't). But I do have a little secret to share.

You'll spend years dreaming about this child, and nine months growing them from a little bean into a real live person. You'll stress and pray and read and buy and obsess along the way. And then at some point, maybe early on, maybe years down the line, you realize the secret.

The secret is that everything you ever needed to know about parenting wasn't in a book or on a blog or in Babies "R" Us.

It was in them. In those giggles, and tummy time, and tiny little hands.

So grow them, love them, and hold them close. And in return, they will teach you exactly how to be the parent they need.

Almost as if it was meant to be.

Acknowledgments

TO MY AGENT Lilly Ghahremani for being with me from the very beginning and always helping me navigate my way along this crazy writing journey. To Seal Press, which has believed in my voice since book #1. I know how lucky I am to have found such a supportive home all those years ago. To my editor, Laura Mazer, for pushing me to be better and always looking out for my books along the way.

To my Moms on the Front Lines (Amy, Brooke, Carrie, Colleen, Dana, Deanna, Deborah, Jen, Jill, Jodi, Karen, Kaysee, Melanie, Michaela, Michelle, Rachel, Sarah B., Sarah G., Stephany, and Tara), for never hesitating to share their deeply personal stories. They bring an immeasurable amount of humor and heart to this book and I'm so grateful that they've trusted me with both.

To the Partners (Becky, Jason, Jeremy, Jonathan, Kevin, Krista, Matt, and Pete), whose unique perspectives offered so much more than I was expecting. Their answers to my questions were thoughtful and sincere and may have made me tear up on more than one occasion.

To my parents, Betty Lou and Dave Dais, who have showed up for my kids in the same way they always showed up for me. I may be biased, but I'd say they are two of the top grandparents in the game.

To Becky Rook, for being my partner on this ride, from positive pregnancy tests to toddler meltdowns in the middle of Target. It hasn't always been easy, but it's always been worth it.

To Vivian Lucia and Daniel Paul, who have grown from a wish, to an ultrasound, to real-live tiny humans who are becoming bigger humans every day. For your hugs, your humor, and your innocence. And for being endlessly entertained by my post-pregnancy flabby belly, "Look, Mommy, it feels like Play-Doh!"

Thank you.

MORE BOOKS BY DAWN DAIS

The Sh!t No One Tells You:
A Guide to Surviving Your Baby's First Year

The Sh!t No One Tells You About Toddlers:
A Guide to Surviving Your Toddler Years

The Sh!t No One Tells You About Baby #2:
A Guide To Surviving Your Growing Family

The Overly Honest Baby Book:
Uncensored Memories from Baby's First Year

The Nonrunner's Marathon Guide for Women:
Get Off Your Butt and On with Your Training

$\mathcal{D}$ AWN DAIS IS a writer, designer, and filmmaker. She lives in Sacramento with her partner, two kids, two dogs, two cats, and the occasional mouse brought home by said cats. She is tired. Stalk Dawn online at www.dawndais.com.

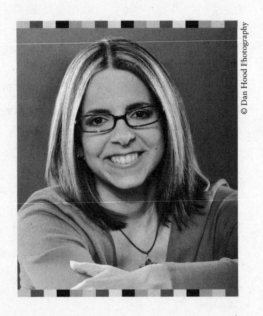

© Dan Hood Photography